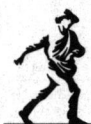

The

BRAIN

Never Sleeps

Why We Dream and
What It Means for Our Health

KAREN
VAN KAMPEN

PUBLISHED BY SIMON & SCHUSTER
New York   Amsterdam/Antwerp   London
Toronto   Sydney/Melbourne   New Delhi

For Dimitri, Alexander, and Claudia

AUTHOR'S NOTE

I BEGAN RESEARCHING AND WRITING "THE DREAM BOOK," AS IT was known in my house, two decades ago. The interviews, dream experiments, research, and my own dreams span space and time. I visited dream labs in Canada and the United States. My manuscript took a transatlantic detour to London, England, where we lived for a couple of years. Coincidentally, our drafty, charming flat was within walking distance of the house where Sigmund Freud spent his last days.

Such a lengthy book project gave me the chance to record and reflect on my dreams during pregnancy and new parenthood and experience how such pivotal life events have the power to shape our dreams. Sleepless nights, the constant whir of our son's rain machine, and nightmares of losing him in a crowd let me witness the effects of poor sleep quality and daytime preoccupations on our dreams. Bookending this are my recent and sometimes turbulent dreams charting the course of planned and unexpected changes in work and in life.

Over many years, I had the opportunity to meet and learn from some of the world's leading dream researchers, some of whom have since passed away. In all possible circumstances, I have connected with the scientists, researchers, and avid dreamers who generously shared their time and expertise to confirm details from our conversations that in some cases date back many years. I've been gifted an appreciation and greater understanding of dreams, this mysterious and often overlooked other realm of existence that is accessible to each of us, for which I am forever grateful.

CONTENTS

The

BRAIN

Never Sleeps

INTRODUCTION

The Art and Science of Dreaming

IN 1932, SALVADOR DALÍ'S *THE PERSISTENCE OF MEMORY* EXHIBITED in New York City. You might know it as *The Melting Clocks* or *Soft Watches*. It's a small piece of art, despite its vastness on canvas and its poster-sized reproductions tacked onto the walls of dorm rooms around the world. The Spanish surrealist artist invites us into his in-between world of reality and fantasy, which he called "hand-painted dream photographs."

In the background, there is a vast blue sky and the craggy cliffs of Mount Pani towering over the coastline of Catalonia, Spain, where Dalí was from. This situates us in this world, even if it's at a distance. The foreground features Dalí's famous soft clocks. He called these the "camembert of time," which were inspired by Dalí musing over a plate of soft French cheese melting in the sun. There is a figure in the middle of the painting. It seems to be a person's profile with the long, feathery lashes of a closed eye, a pointed, beak-like nose, and open mouth. Is it Dalí? Is he asleep? Could this all be a dream?

It's a mix of permanence and impermanence, of light and shadows, of this world and another. Dalí was tormented by a fear of insects and sensations of imaginary bugs crawling along his skin. On the back of a pocket watch, there is a swarm of ants, which Dalí often used to represent death and destruction. Here, time decays in the sun. It's a timeless, boundless place. The surreal and the real are brought to life with the same razor-sharp attention to detail, making the landscape of his childhood just as real as his dreamscape. The familiar and recognizable are juxtaposed with the fantastical and seemingly impossible. It's a trick of the eye, which creates confusion and wonder. Objects seem to hide in plain sight. As with all of Dalí's works, the longer you look at it, the more you see. And the more you see, the more you feel. Much like a dream.

In the early 1920s while studying art in Madrid, Dalí discovered the writing of Sigmund Freud, known as the father of dreams. For Dalí, *The Interpretation of Dreams* was "one of the capital discoveries of my life," he wrote. "I was seized with a real vice of self-interpretation, not only of my dreams but of everything that happened to me."[1] At the same time, Dalí was drawn to the surrealists, artists and writers in Paris who brought the subconscious to life on the canvas and on the page. It was a time of artistic transformation and discovery. Dalí developed his surrealist style, bridging the waking and dreaming worlds with his magical dreamscapes.

In the early 1930s, Dalí crafted his "paranoiac critical" method. He invoked a state of paranoia to tap into the subconscious and explore the concept of identity, using hallucinations as inspiration for his art. He took bizarre found objects in his subconscious and brought them to life on canvas through strange juxtapositions, hidden or overlayed images, and optical illusions. He wanted to "materialize the images of concrete irrationality."[2] Surrealists explored the "surreality" of subjective experiences, and Dalí found that dreams offered unique personal experiences, and as inspiration.

There were many ways that he tapped into the creativity of his dreams. Possibly the most famous is his "slumber with a key" method. Think of it as a power nap. Here's how it works. Imagine Dalí with his characteristic mustache, which lengthened and twisted upward over the years, sitting in a "bony armchair, preferably of Spanish style," which he recommended. With his head tipped back, his hands suspended midair, below the arms of the chair. In his left hand, he held a key "delicately pressed between the extremities of the thumb and forefinger."[3] Underneath the suspended key was a plate. The moment Dalí fell asleep, floating between this world and dreams, he let go of the key, which fell onto the plate, waking him up. In the magical first moments of sleep, Dalí discovered a wild montage of images for his art. His inner self was his muse.

In recent years, scientists have shown physiologically what Dalí knew to be true: sleep onset, when we first fall asleep, is a "creative sweet spot" that lets us make unexpected and original connections among abstract ideas.[4] For Dalí, and for the dreamer in all of us, the science facilitates the art of dreaming.

A Traveler's Guide to Dreams

When I try to trace back my fascination with dreams, a certain memory pops into my head. I was nine years old, sitting in the kitchen of my childhood home in Oshawa, Ontario, that's about an hour's drive from Toronto. My feet snaked around the legs of a creaky wooden chair. My parents hadn't renovated the kitchen yet, so I was surrounded by faded blue-flowered wallpaper. I pulled my long hair off my face and tilted my head back. Our German shepherds Pepper and Spice circled the room, then paused to take a closer look. My father wrestled with a tangle of colourful wires and a pot of sticky white paste. He consulted an official-looking book, then glanced back at me over the large round rims of his glasses, determining where to place the electrodes.

My dad, Murray Moffat, is a sleep doctor. In 1982, he opened one of the first independent sleep laboratories in Canada. He became interested in sleep while working as a coroner. When he was called to a site, he would sometimes find a person in bed or on the couch, having died inexplicably in their sleep. It often appeared to be a coronary, but why, he wondered, were so many people having heart attacks in the night? At the time, sleep studies were mostly run in universities and hospitals, and my dad remembers them being performed in the halls of a Toronto psychiatric institute. He decided to set up a facility dedicated to diagnosing and treating sleep disorders.

As a kid, I imagined my childhood home as its own kind of sleep lab. The bedrooms had blackout blinds and mattresses with just the right firmness. At night, the temperature was a cool 68 degrees. Around the house, there were stacks of the journal *Sleep* and balls of knotted electrodes that my dad was always repairing for his actual sleep lab. It was a house wired for sleep and I was my dad's first lab "assistant." In our kitchen, he would hook me up with electrodes to practice the patient set-up and I'd help him string cables throughout the house, testing the computer networks for his lab. I watched him flip through test sleep records, each a paper tower of one thousand pages, as he scanned for renegade sleep patterns inked onto an accordion of crisp white paper.

Sometimes we would drive into Toronto, where he was setting up his sleep lab at the Medical Arts Building on Bloor Street. It had three bedrooms where his patients would soon sleep. Each headboard had an emerald-green box the electrodes were plugged into, and the bedrooms were soundproof. All you could hear was the soothing whir of cool air.

At the other end of a skinny hallway was the control area that housed three mammoth polysomnography (PSG) machines. Each had a shiny, stainless steel frame and a panel of knobs and switches that I resisted flicking back and forth for fear of shutting down the entire lab. Blank sleep records were fed into the PSGs, which inked the pages with scribbling pens. As patients slept, electrodes would send signals to the machines, recording their brain activity, movement, and breathing. I envisioned the lab as a cross between a hotel, with fresh sheets and towels, and a top-secret government facility tracking the secrets of the night.

I was there so my dad could make sure all the equipment worked properly. My father would watch the controls as I blinked and breathed in and out. Then he would leave me to do what I did best: sleep. Within minutes, my dreaming brain would transport me from the small bedroom to strange and unexpected places.

I still remember sitting next to my dad as he took me through my sleep record. He flipped through the accordion of crisp pages so fast that it seemed like the squiggly lines that had tracked my brain activity, breathing, and eye movement were moving. It reminded me of my homemade flip books of moving images, of flying birds and crashing waves.

Sleep and dreams have always been comforting to me. When I was a kid, I would fall asleep to escape bad turbulence on a flight or snowstorms as we drove across the Prairies to visit family. I would even fall asleep if I was bored. In dreams, there was so much to investigate and explore. I loved the freedom of letting my mind wander and pursue whatever wild thoughts I could imagine, unrestrained by the demands and distractions of the day. Dreaming was its own kind of freedom of thought and expression.

I grew up thinking and learning about sleep. It was the analog world of the eighties, long before sleep became its own industry with wearables and trending sleep hacks. When I was a kid, my parents dragged me and my brother across the States to see what other labs were doing. I moved on from my stint as a lab assistant, taking on a variety of jobs at the sleep lab. In high school and university, I did data entry and organized storage units of paper records. It was years before sleep records went digital, and we stored the paper records from the six-bed lab for ten years, which generated skyscraper-worthy stacks of paper.

One summer, my friend Katie Rodgers worked with me at the lab. One of our jobs was to transport the sleep records to storage units. We used to fill a Jeep with paper records until the old vehicle sagged at the back. Then we'd drive the country roads from the lab to the storage facility. I'll never forget the time that we were driving along, singing to Jane's Addiction, when I noticed a breeze coming from behind us. The hatch had sprung open, and I watched in my rearview mirror as thousands of pages fanned out into the night sky. It was the last run of the day. With only the Jeep's headlights to guide us, we ran across the country road, chasing after flying pages, dipping into gullies and sifting through weeds and wild grass to grab the paper chains of records. We rolled up the pages, stuffed it all into the Jeep and filled the storage unit with gigantic balls of paper. Somehow, we were able to retrieve every last record.

In later years, I worked with doctors, nurses, and sleep technicians at the lab. I went on to oversee daytime operations and helped develop virtual sleep services before wearable sleep technology went mainstream. As a writer, I believe in the power of accessible, trustworthy information to improve our health and well-being. I'm passionate about prioritizing sleep in our busy lives and spreading the word about its importance in our physical and mental health.

The nine-year-old kid in me is still in complete wonder of the dreams that sleep offers. I'm as fascinated by the fantasy as by the reality of dreams; the fictions our dreaming brain creates and the real moments on which it shines a spotlight.

A couple of years ago, I came across a paper by Rubin Naiman called "Dreamless: The Silent Epidemic of REM Sleep Loss." I learned that we are as dream deprived as we are sleep deprived, and our REM dream loss is harming our physical and mental health. It made sense that if we weren't getting enough sleep, then we weren't having enough dreams. The idea of a dream deprived society shifted my focus back to dreams. Why, I wanted to know, are dreams important in their own right? Why do dreams matter, and what benefits are we missing out on if we are depriving ourselves of dreams? Naiman explained that our REM dream loss is harming our health and well-being. To make matters worse, we are in denial of the deleterious effects of REM dream loss.

How, I wondered, did we get here? Why don't we pay more attention to our dreams? In our sleep-deprived society, dreams can be hard to come by. I've had my fair share of sleepless nights because of illness and puzzling bouts of insomnia, a sick child, or a frightened puppy. I thought about how difficult it is to ponder our dreams when we're in survival mode, trying to snatch whatever sleep we can get. I thought of another possible contributing factor: dreams have a bit of an image problem. As several dream researchers told me, dreams still carry psychoanalytic baggage from the time of Sigmund Freud, who believed that dreams are unfulfilled repressed wishes. The neuroscience of dreams offers another side of the debate over the meaning of dreams, focusing on the neural mechanisms of the dreaming process.

In this accelerated world, many of us don't stop and think about our dreams, as if they were fictions unrelated to us, the ones who created them. "Today, too many of us view dreams the way we do stars—they emerge nightly and seem magnificent, but are far too distant to be of any relevance in our lives," wrote Naiman.[5]

This reignited my fascination with dreams. I had a big picture understanding of why we dream, which left many unanswered questions. Why, I wondered, do we spend so much time and energy to create such complex dream stories? Wouldn't a simple plot line suffice? How are dreams connected to our waking lives and, as a result, our mental health? When I'm preoccupied or worried, my concerns often show up in my dreams in strange and bizarre ways. But what insights lay beyond my personal dream experiences and general reading on dreams? I wanted to dig deeper into the research. I was curious to understand how dreams can gauge our current state of mind and then change along with our psychological well-being. Above all, I wanted to learn how we can use our dreams to improve our mental health. I had many questions to investigate and expand my thinking, which set me off on this journey through dreamland.

This is a book about the art and the science of dreaming. It's about how dreams are built, why we dream, and how we can use our dreams in everyday life. It's about the intrinsic connection between dreams and our well-being. Dreams illuminate our state of mind, from everyday worries and preoccupations to struggles with our mental health. Dreams reveal what matters most to us and what remains unsettled in our lives. During times of crisis, dreams tell the story.

This is the story of my exploration of the dark side of the mind that is often dismissed or forgotten. We spend a large amount of our waking hours daydreaming and a third of our lives asleep. We think of ourselves as rational and analytic. Yet above all, we are dreamers. We spend a lot of our time imagining and planning, with our minds elsewhere. In dreams, we are free thinkers who pursue the impossible. Yet many of us don't pay much attention to our dreams. We are busy thinking every moment of our lives, whether it's waking or dreaming thoughts that swirl around our heads. *The Brain Never Sleeps* investigates dreaming as part of this twenty-four-hour loop.

It examines many facets of dreaming, from the psychology to the neuroscience of dreams, and weaves scientific findings with personal experiences. Through interviews, research, and dreams that span two decades, I share what I learned about the art and science of dreaming, including why dreams matter and how we can reclaim this other realm of thought and experience.

I begin my tour through dreamland with Sigmund Freud as my guide. It has been well over a century since Freud published *The Interpretation of Dreams*, and the debate continues over the meaning and nonsense of dreams. I discover that it isn't an either-or situation with a dream being a mental junkyard or a psychological dig just waiting for the archaeologist in us to uncover its meaning. Dreams by their very nature are about possibility, offering many facets and complexities to explore. I dig up early dream experiments and chart the course of some trailblazing dream researchers whose work is often overshadowed by Freud. These pioneers in dream science experimented with their own dreams, proposing some of the major dream theories that are still studied today.

Next, I examine how dreams are made. I look at the mental mechanics of the dreaming brain to understand why our thoughts and experiences are so different in dreams. As we travel through a night of sleep, parts of the brain quiet down while other areas hum with activity. At certain points, different parts of our brain are as active as when we are awake. I learn how the dreaming brain works in a different mode, which changes how we think, behave, and imagine what is possible. We might fly through the air and convince ourselves it's really happening. Our dreams are as real to us as our waking experiences. For some of us, the nightly journey doesn't go so smoothly. REM behaviour disorder is a rare kind of sleep disorder that has people act out their dreams, sometimes with devastating and even fatal consequences.

While dreams aren't replays of waking life, they illuminate our preoccupations and worries that we are so skilled at avoiding during the day, from difficult conversations to facing our darkest fears or coping with many kinds of loss. Dreams offer new perspectives on ourselves and others. As I learned about the intrinsic connection between dreams and our mental health, I kept coming back to Bessel van der Kolk's *The Body Keeps the Score*. The book had opened up a new way of thinking for me on how we carry and process trauma. It made me think about how dreams know the score, revealing our true state of mind.

Dreams indicate how we are feeling and coping at the moment. They are a kind of natural warning system, signaling when to attend to our mental health. We can learn a lot from our dreams simply by paying attention to recurrent themes and unresolved issues. This highlights what is emotionally important to us and needs our attention. In speaking with scientists, I discover that we can be a poor judge of our level of stress and how it's affecting us biologically. Sometimes dreams tell a different story than the one we are telling ourselves. If we are struggling during the day, there is a good chance this will play out in our dreams.

Our everyday worries and preoccupations along with mental health struggles often become the focus of our dreams. About 50 percent to 70 percent of people with post-traumatic stress disorder (PTSD) suffer from recurrent nightmares, which can cause severe distress at night and during the day and sometimes continue for decades. Negative recurrent dreams can be distressing, although on a much milder scale, as we ruminate over unresolved thoughts, feelings, and situations. Upsetting dreams can follow us into the next day, creating a continuum of negative waking and dreaming thoughts.

I discover there is a positive side to this difficult dream work. Researchers have found that positive well-being, specifically peace of mind, can lead to positive dreams. So if we are able to create a calm mindset during the day, this might also improve our dream life. During the night, dreams offer a safe space to process difficult emotions. I find there are effective techniques to rescript nightmares and change our reactions to them. In this way, it makes each of us an empowered dreamer.

This brings me to the fundamental question that researchers have been exploring for more than a century: Why do we dream? I speak with many scientists to gain their different perspectives, which leads me to in-sleep as well as post-sleep effects of dreams. Does the work happen when we are asleep, and we benefit even if we don't remember our dreams? One idea is that we dream to strengthen and integrate memories into our existing catalogue of experience and knowledge. Another theory suggests that a dream is a nightly therapy session that helps us process emotional memories. Or could the value of dreams be found when we reflect on them in the morning?

In speaking with scientists, physicians, and psychologists, I've found that beyond their possible functions are the many ways we can use dreams in our everyday life. I try some of my own dream experiments, testing different tools and techniques to make the most out of my dreams. I use an AI dream analysis tool to interpret one of my dreams using Freudian and Jungian modes and then sit down with a psychologist to understand the results. I participate in my first "dream salon" where some friends, avid dreamers, and researchers help me figure out a particularly strange dream while an artist brings my dream to life. I talk to people who have experienced a certain kind of "big dream," as Carl Jung called it, that transformed their lives. I discover the subtle revelations of little dreams from everyday life that can inspire big change.

I travel to the next frontier in dreaming where I meet dream engineers who are using technology to guide our dreams. I speak with a graduate student and her undergraduate subject who one January morning in Evanston, Illinois, opened the lines of communication between the waking and dreaming worlds. She asked the sleeping undergrad a math problem, and he answered with staccato left-right, left-right eye movements behind closed lids. Along the way, I gather tips and techniques on how to make the most of our dreams. I have shared some of these in the Dreamer's Toolkit at the back of the book.

Finally, I try an at-home dream experiment to guide my dreams during sleep onset, those first few minutes of sleep where Dalí found inspiration. The surrealist artist was in his late twenties when he painted *The Persistence of Memory*, a tiny canvas just over nine by thirteen inches that is like a portal into his vast dreamscape. It sold for $250. A few years later, it was donated to the Museum of Modern Art, where it is still on display.

I explore the physiology of the universal dream phenomenon and the psychology of this personal experience. On my tour of the dream world, I discover why dreams matter, how they are connected to our mental health, and ways we can use them to improve our waking and dreaming lives. Let's dream big.

Chapter One

THE FREUD EFFECT

WHEN I LIVED IN LONDON SOME YEARS AGO, I USED TO PASS A blackened bronze statue on my daily walk to Finchley Road, a busy, dismal, yet useful thoroughfare teeming with shops and amenities in northwest London. On overcast days, the statue was dull and mute. When it poured, rained, or drizzled, in typical London fashion, heavy raindrops accumulated on the tip of the figure's nose, plopping into a puddle in his lap. On those magical sunny days when the ceiling of clouds was lifted from the city, revealing a big blue sky, the statue shone. But I was oblivious to all of this. I'd just had a baby, and I bumped my stroller along the cobblestone streets of my new neighbourhood, navigating my way through the dense and disorienting fog of sleeplessness.

One day my husband joined me on my trek to the shops. We took the shortcut to Waitrose, meandering along narrow backstreets, past the local wine store, pharmacy, and café. Rounding the corner toward Finchley Road, Dimitri stopped and looked up. Staring down at us was the statue of a balding, bearded man with raised, inquisitive eyebrows, clad in a distinguished three-piece suit. He sat with his hands perched on his hips, leaning forward toward the road, casting a watchful gaze on the passing crowd.

"Hey, it's Freud," said Dimitri.

Staring down at me was the father of psychoanalysis, the Austrian neurologist who popularized dream interpretation and the man forever known to proclaim that dreams are the attempted fulfillment of our repressed wishes. I stood there, wide-eyed, as if waking up to this new sight. With my line of vision raised from the stroller, I noticed a sign pointing to the Freud Museum around the next corner. For almost half a year, I'd been living only a few blocks away from the house where Freud had spent his last days.

How, you might wonder, could I have been so unaware? For starters, I was a new mother living thousands of miles away from family and friends. When Alexander was eight weeks old, Dimitri and I packed up our worldly belongings, which at the time consisted mostly of Ikea furniture and bright, loud baby toys, along with boxes of research for this book, which began many years ago. We moved from Toronto to north London's Belsize Park, a leafy neighbourhood with a charming village vibe, teeming with buggies, dogs, and local shops along winding cobblestone streets. I soon found that I was living a cruel irony. My dad is a sleep doctor who opened one of the first independent sleep laboratories in Canada when I was a kid. Let's just say that we talked about the importance of sleep. A lot. My newborn son decided that he didn't like to sleep at night. And then there was the kicker: I was writing a book on dreams. I'm sure Freud would've had something to say about this.

The world around me was dreamlike, seeming both unknown and familiar. I'd visited London over the years, so there was a familiarity to the city. I had memories of long walks through Hyde Park, going treasure hunting among the stalls of Camden Market, and cheering on street performers doing magic tricks, acrobatics, and singing opera from the cobblestones of Covent Garden. Yet I was so sleep-deprived that I was seeing things through a different lens. I was operating in another mode, much like a dream, which shaped how I experienced the world around me. I remembered only snippets of a day's worth of memories. No wonder I'd gone months without noticing Freud staring down at me.

But I didn't need a statue to feel Freud's presence. He was one of the twentieth century's most influential thinkers. He remains engrained in our culture and collective psyche. While Freud was not the first to study dreams, his work propelled dream research into the next century. To this day, the mere mention of his name can spark heated debate. Some would say that dream research is still weighed down by psychoanalytic baggage. And while some of Freud's ideas are outdated and have been debunked by scientists, several of his theories laid the groundwork for research that continues to this day. It's been more than 125 years since Freud published *The Interpretation of Dreams*, and this great, controversial figure continues to be quoted by students, scientists, and avid dreamers. Even grade-schoolers know who Freud is. He laid down the royal road to the enigmatic unconscious mind. So I decided that I'd better pay a visit to Freud's last home and refuge, the epicenter of dream analysis.

The House of Dreams

TWENTY MARESFIELD GARDENS IS a stately, red brick house with three floors of white framed windows, impeccably trimmed hedges, and a blossoming almond tree that Freud used to admire. The gloriously sunny spring day I was there many years ago, Bobby, the museum's elderly guard dog, dozed underneath its canopy of white flowers, ignoring me as I walked along the stone path and through the front door. Inside, the foyer was spacious and elegant, with a spiral staircase and polished wooden floors. To my right I found a narrow doorway leading to a dark, still room that smelled of old books, having lost the scent of Freud's beloved cigars.

This was Freud's study where he wrote and saw patients between 1938 and 1939 during the last year of his life. In the late thirties, as the Nazis overtook Austria, Freud knew he was in grave danger. He was among the Jewish writers whose books were burned by the Germans. So he took refuge in London, living his final year in exile. Comparing his family's living conditions in Vienna to London, Freud wrote in his diary that they went from "poverty to white bread."[1]

His study was spacious and grand, about five times the size of my own writing space. It spanned the length of the house and had tall windows on either end, overlooking the front and back yards. Dark bookshelves filled with leather-bound volumes reached the high ceiling. A four-step wooden ladder stood in front of the shelves, its edges rounded and worn from Freud's dress shoes climbing in search of hard-to-reach books.

If the burgundy velvet drapes were open, I could have peered into the lush back garden where Freud liked to relax on a swinging lounge, shaded by its canopy. He would take his papers into the backyard and read with his feet up, pausing to chat with visitors. Near the back window, I found his famous analyst's couch, draped in a once-colourful rug, its royal blue, plum, and cream patterns now faded and worn. I imagined his patients with their heads propped against two now-flattened pillows, giving detailed accounts of their dreams during therapy sessions. Freud would listen from his forest-green velvet tub chair at the head of the couch, out of his patients' sight, encouraging them to let their minds wander.

In the late 1800s, Freud unveiled psychoanalysis, a psychotherapy technique that explores the conscious and unconscious mind in order to uncover and analyze people's fantasies and fears. To unveil what was tearing at people's psyches, Freud devised the method of free association, asking them to relay whatever was on their minds, regardless of how silly or inconsequential these thoughts may have seemed. Yet he found that there were limits to what the conscious mind revealed. Freud believed that dreams harbour our fundamental instincts, including sexuality, aggression, and self-love. Some of our instincts are too painful, embarrassing, or damning for our fragile conscious to bear, so they are held captive by our unconscious. Freud used dream interpretation to analyze and free our instincts and wishes, including those we repress.

While Freud studied the dreams of patients, colleagues, and friends, his regular subject was himself. He'd been fascinated by dreams since he was a boy, and had always been an avid dreamer, observing and recording his nightly fictions in a journal. With *The Interpretation of Dreams*, Freud wanted to show how his dream interpretation methods could be used to unearth the layered meanings of dreams.

According to Freud, there are two types of dream content to analyze. There is the manifest content, which is what we recall when we wake up. This includes what Freud described as "day residue," references or fragments of events from the previous day. The manifest content isn't supposed to make sense on its own. Freud believed that the real meaning of a dream could be found in its latent content, the subterranean layer of a dream that lies beneath its surface. This includes our disguised wishes and instincts. Reflecting on our personal associations, experiences, and emotions, we can interpret the latent content of our dreams and discover hidden meanings.

Freud is famous for seeing the erotic in life's seemingly ordinary objects. "The majority of dream-symbols serve to represent persons, parts of the body and activities invested with erotic interest," wrote Freud in a 1911 addition to *On Dreams*, a condensed version of *The Interpretation of Dreams*. "Sharp weapons, long and stiff objects, such as tree-trunks and sticks, stand for the male genitals; while cupboards, boxes, carriages or ovens may represent the uterus." Yet Freud didn't believe that all of our wishes are sexually charged. He felt that we are motivated by other instincts, including aggression and narcissism.

Freud devised the idea that dreams are the attempted fulfillment of a wish by analyzing one of his own dreams known as Irma's Injection. In the dream, Freud was at a large gathering where he saw his patient Irma. They chatted about her health, and he announced rather bluntly that if she was still in pain, it was her fault. Irma told Freud that he had no idea of her physical suffering. He was startled by her pale and puffy complexion. On closer examination, he discovered that she had an infection, and realized it was from an injection that had been administered by one of Freud's physician friends who used an unclean syringe.

Freud reflected on his dream. "I am refusing to be blamed for all the pain she still has," he wrote. "If it is Irma's own fault it cannot be mine. Is the intention of the dream to be sought for in this direction?"[2] Freud wondered if he wished to be innocent of his patient's ill health. This spiraled into Freud's concerns over the health of his wife, his competency as a physician, and the memory of his daughter's illness. The dream's layers of meaning were like the thin, transparent skin of an onion that Freud peeled back to expose one hidden truth after another.

One night while living in London, I dreamt that I was sitting on the edge of my bed, unable to quiet my shaking hands as I called the police to report my husband missing. Dimitri had been gone for days and Alexander wouldn't stop crying. I gathered our family and friends to search the city, but we couldn't find him anywhere. When my son's hungry cries woke me up, I looked over to find Dimitri, sleeping soundly beside me. He had worked late for several weeks, getting home long after I'd gone to bed. So it made sense that he went missing in my dream. I wasn't afraid that he would actually disappear. I just wished that he could be around more.

About the same time, I dreamt of my teeth slowly falling out, one by one, and in this recurrent dream within a dream, my sleeping self woke up choking on bits of enamel. I've discovered that teeth dreams are common. One study found that 39 percent of subjects had dreamt of teeth while 16.2 percent of subjects had recurrent dreams about their teeth rotting, breaking, or falling out.[3] Is there a psychological reason for my teeth dreams? I think it's more likely because I grind my teeth when I'm stressed. In fact, a recent study found that teeth dreams are related to dental irritation.[4] So if we've got tension in our jaw, we might incorporate this sensation into our dreams.

Where does our mind find the content for our dreams? According to Freud, there are two main sources: memories from our past, which include emotions and experiences from our childhood, as well as "day residue" of past events, particularly from the previous day. Shortly after getting engaged to Martha, Freud wrote to her about his dreams, which he described as unruly. Freud noticed that he dreamt of themes that he touched on briefly in his waking life before moving on. Scientists have since advanced the concept of day residue and shown that we carry waking preoccupations and concerns into our dreams, shining a spotlight on what's important to us.

To mine our dreams for meaning, Freud believed that we must use mental tools like condensation and displacement. Condensation occurs when a variety of thoughts, emotions, or associations conjures one dream image or element. This creates many meanings from one image. Displacement happens when the emotions attached to a certain event or person are transferred, or displaced, to something completely unrelated that may be less threatening or a more acceptable target for those emotions—anger, for example. Let's say someone had an argument with their partner that left them unsettled. Maybe in their dream, they cracked their knee against a large dresser and screamed at the piece of furniture, taking their anger out on the inanimate object.

Artifacts of the Night

STANDING IN THE SHADOWS of his dimly lit study, I imagined Freud pondering his dream theories at his desk, which was set back from the window so the sun wouldn't shine directly onto his work. Freud was right-handed, and this positioning ensured the light would stream across his left shoulder. The desk looked small in the middle of the large room that reflected the atmosphere of his study in Vienna. Freud described his new house as spacious, comfortable, and light, despite its drafty sash windows that let in bone-chilling London air. But it wasn't home until he was able to reclaim his precious antiquities collection. When he escaped the Nazis, Freud was forced to leave his treasured objects in Vienna. After many agonizing months, the Germans released his things. When they arrived at Maresfield Gardens, he wrote in his diary that he was finally "free of the Nazis."[5]

Freud collected more than two thousand statues, busts, reliefs, and prints from Rome, Egypt, and Greece. He was fascinated by ancient civilizations and the things that people worshipped and feared, the spirits and gods that appeared in their dreams and occupied their waking thoughts. Just as he studied dreams that the conscious mind had repressed, he studied objects that people had found after they had been buried and lost for years. And with every new artifact, he dug up another mystery of humanity. Freud said to one of his patients that the psychoanalyst, like the archaeologist, must uncover layer upon layer of a patient's psyche to discover the most valuable treasures.

As I studied the crowded row of statuettes on his desk, I imagined the multitude of gazes staring back at him while he worked. It's been said that Freud's state of mind was reflected in the objects on his desk. *A Guide to the Freud Museum* describes them as his tools of thought and the kitchen utensils of his imagination. As I stared at his beloved antiquities collection, I imagined peering into Freud's inner self. This is the thread that runs through his collection. The thread is Freud's unconscious, which is revealed in three dimensions.[6]

The object that took centre stage was a bronze Roman statuette of Athena, which had been smuggled out of Vienna by his friend Princess Marie Bonaparte, the great-grandniece of French Emperor Napoleon. The goddess of wisdom and war had a breastplate adorned with Medusa's head. Her arm was raised, ready to throw her spear, which was missing from her hand. Among the row of figures was the famous sphinx from fifth century BC. It was half-lion, half-woman, with an animal's large paws and strong body coupled with pointy breasts and a soft, feminine face. It's thought that the statue was the inspiration for Freud's Oedipus Complex, his psychoanalytic theory based on the Greek myth of Oedipus, who unwittingly married his mother and killed his father.

Freud was grief stricken after his father died in 1896. Retreating inwards, he was hit by this "truth": that we love and adore our parent of the opposite sex while hating our parent of the same sex. Freud said to his friend and confidant Wilhelm Fliess, "I have found, in my own case too, [the phenomenon of] being in love with my mother and jealous of my father, and I now consider it a universal event in early childhood."[7] According to Freud, we must resolve this inner struggle that surfaces during childhood if we are to become well-adjusted adults.

Writing his iconic dream book was personally meaningful to Freud as he shared his dreams and intimate details of his personal life. Many scientists scoffed at his psychological theory of dreaming, dismissing his book that was written for the masses. Freud didn't turn to psychoanalysis because he dismissed brain science. He was trained as a neurologist by some of the best brain scientists of the time, which is often missing from his story. There were things that the brain simply couldn't explain. It's hard to believe that one of the most influential and quoted books sold only 351 copies in its first six years of publication.[8]

Freud published *The Interpretation of Dreams* in 1900, signaling the beginning of a new and exciting century of dream research. Yet there were many groundbreaking discoveries that foreshadowed some of Freud's prominent dream theories. In the mid-1800s, several researchers conducted experiments, often using their own dreams as evidence. These trailblazers advanced dream research, questioning the possibilities and boundaries of the dreaming mind. While some of their discoveries led to dream theories that are still recognized today, these curious scientists and passionate dreamers are often overshadowed by Freud. Here are some of their stories.

Field Notes from Dreamland

IN 1861, ALFRED MAURY, a librarian, professor of history at Collège de France, and scholar of dreams, published *Le Sommeil et les Rêves* (Sleep and Dreams), which chronicled his own dreams and observations of the universal dreaming experience. For many years, Maury recorded his dreams in meticulous detail to try and unravel the mysteries of the dreaming mind and how it creates our nightly musings. To analyze his dreams when they were still fresh in his mind, Maury had someone wake him throughout the night. "Awoken with a start, the memory of the dream from which I have been torn away is still present in my mind, in its pristine freshness. . . . I consign these observations to a notebook, in the same way as a doctor keeps case notes."[9]

Maury noted how our dreaming mind combines recent and distant memories to create a cohesive narrative. In one dream, he travelled up and down the streets of New York City with a friend. When he awoke, Maury had a clear picture of the city in his mind. In particular, he envisioned a square within New York. He had seen a print of New York in the window of a shop. So he returned to the shop to find the image of New York. Yet the panoramic view prevented him from identifying the square from his dream. Racking his brain, he remembered a drawing of a square in Mexico City. Later, Maury happened upon the image of the drawing in a book. Maury realized that he had combined the remembered image from Mexico City with his imaginings of New York, a place he had never visited.

Through years of self-observation, Maury determined that dreams are a combination of the recognizable and the bizarre. He believed that moments from our lifetime catalogues of thoughts, experiences, and knowledge find their way into our dreams, including lost memories that can resurface from our childhood. Yet at the same time, he identified the fantastical nature of dreams as we mix recognizable memories with imaginary scenarios, creating original combinations. He believed in the automatic workings of the dreaming mind to create unique associations among our waking experiences.

Maury's famous "guillotine dream" illustrates how our mind combines real and imagined knowledge and experiences to create a cohesive story. It occurred one night when Maury was sick and his mother was taking care of him. In his dream, Maury was transported back to the Reign of Terror, a brutally violent period in France during the late 1700s in which thousands of people were executed by the guillotine. Maury dreamt that he was condemned to death and ushered onto the scaffold, where his head was placed under the guillotine blade. A large crowd of people watched the blade fall. Maury experienced the sensation of his head being severed from his body. He bolted awake to discover that the headboard had fallen and hit the back of his neck where a guillotine blade would have struck.[10]

Freud had his own analysis of Maury's guillotine dream that he described in *The Interpretation of Dreams*. Freud believed that Maury's dream was neither random nor by coincidence. Maury was a boy haunted by the French Revolution, and his guillotine dream revealed clues about his psychological state.[11] At the same time, it raised the question of how such a rich, detailed narrative could be dreamt in the time between Maury being hit by his headboard and being woken by the painful sensation. This led to a long-held belief that dreams are an almost instantaneous experience.

In the 1850s, Maury experimented with his own dreams to explore how external stimuli can shape our dream stories. While Maury slept, his assistant dripped water onto his forehead, tickled his nose and mouth with a feather, and placed a bottle of cologne under his nose. In one instance, the assistant hit tweezers against a pair of scissors, creating a soft ringing. That night, Maury dreamt of alarm bells ringing to indicate a revolution breaking out, which may have been connected to his memory of the 1848 Paris Revolution. When a hot iron was placed near Maury, he dreamt that people broke into his house and put his feet over the fire, demanding he tell them where he kept his money.[12]

At the time, a distinguished French scientist and professor from the Collège du France was conducting his own personal study of dreams. Growing up in Paris, Marie-Jean-Léon d'Hervey de Saint-Denys began recording his dreams at the age of thirteen. One day, he decided to take the memories of a vivid dream and create a sketch to accompany the description. "Soon I had a special album, where the representation of each scene and figure was accompanied by a clarification," he wrote at the beginning of *Les Rêves et les Moyens de les Diriger: Observations Pratiques* (Dreams and the Ways to Guide Them: Practical Observations). The groundbreaking book, which was initially published anonymously, provides a self-analysis of Saint-Denys's dream stories as well as the common experience of dreaming. Saint-Denys had a wealth of dream stories to analyze. Over five years and 1,946 nights, he created a dream diary with vivid descriptions and coloured illustrations. By creating this diary, he discovered that the act of contemplating and recording his dreams increased his dream recall.

In *Les Rêves*, Saint-Denys described the imprint of our waking lives on our dreams, including our experiences as well as our concerns. Dreams create visual narratives out of the "objects which occupy our thoughts."[13] Many of our dream images stem from long forgotten memories or reminiscences that are reshaped by our imagination. He used the example of a deceased person coming alive in a dream. Our catalogue of memories, remembered and forgotten, are what he called cliché-memories, with cliché being a photographic plate. Just as a photographer collects drawers of negatives of images that may become unrecognizable or possibly even forgotten over time, with so many other images being seen, we too may forget our lifetime collections of memories that "may be hidden in the unfathomable depths of the brain where the cliché-memories are infinitely storing every moment of our lives, and mostly without our knowledge."[14]

Images of two ideas may appear in a dream at the same time, superimposing one image onto the other. Saint-Denys compared this to inserting two glass plates into a lantern. The images combine, either side by side or one on top of the other, and appear simultaneously as one image. If the two images are of people, this may result in a combined figure with two faces and four legs. One night, Saint-Denys dreamt of the grand sphinx on display at the gate of the Tuileries in Paris. The sphinx was from Sebastopol (Sevastopol), located on the southwest coast of the Crimea where an eleven-month siege took place to occupy the port during the Crimean War. The image of this sphinx evoked an image of Saint-Denys's friend who died in the Crimean War. At the same time, Saint-Denys imagined other sphinxes from ruins in Egypt. This conjured an image of Saint-Denys visiting the Egyptian ruins with his friend who had passed away several years earlier.[15] This superimposition of images is akin to Freud's method of condensation in which an idea or object within a dream represents several concepts or associations.

According to Saint-Denys, another way dream images combine is by transferring the qualities of one object to another in a process he called abstraction. In Les Rêves, he described an emaciated horse and the strings of a horse-drawn carriage that showed up in one of his dreams. This carriage might have reminded Saint-Denys of a wagon belonging to a farmer he had seen earlier. The emaciated quality of the horse may be transferred to the farmer, creating a dream image of a weak, feeble farmer.[16] Saint-Denys's idea of abstraction is akin to Freud's theory of displacement in which emotions or characteristics of one person are displaced and transferred into another.

Like Maury, Saint-Denys was curious if external stimuli could appear in our dreams. He conducted dream experiments to explore how sensory experiences can be connected to thoughts, and how memories of these thoughts can influence our dreams. Testing out the power of smell to create dream-worthy memories, Saint-Denys purchased a vial of perfume that was sold to him as one of the most lovely and pleasing scents. With the vial closed tight, he travelled to Vivarais, where he stayed for two weeks with the family of a friend. While he was there, Saint-Denys used the perfume constantly, even dousing his handkerchief in the fragrant scent "despite the objections and jokes which this research caused in my immediate environment."[17]

Ready to be returned home, the vial was sealed tightly, and it remained untouched in a drawer for a couple of months. Then Saint-Denys gave the vial to a servant, asking him to shake a few drops onto his pillow one night without warning Saint-Denys when this would happen. For ten days, he didn't dream of his trip to Vivarais in the southeast of France along the river Rhône. Then one night, he dreamt of a place that he'd once lived for a year. Images of mountains and large chestnut trees appeared in his dream. It was Aubenas in the Rhône Valley in Southern France. Saint-Denys awoke to find that his servant had sprinkled the perfume onto his pillow. He had inhaled the scent while he dreamt. Then Saint-Denys experimented with two scents on his pillow. The one that he used in Vivarais and another that he'd doused his handkerchief with when he worked in a painter's studio. The experiment was repeated several times. It resulted in Saint-Denys dreaming of being in a mountain setting as he watched a painter recreate a beautiful scene on canvas.[18]

Saint-Denys's most impressive feat in shaping his dreams was to control them from within, which is known as lucid dreaming. The first step in becoming lucid is to gain awareness of the dream state. Dreamers can then work on gaining control over their actions as well as the dreamscape through which they navigate. Saint-Denys called this an awareness of his "true situation." He was a skilled lucid dreamer who shared detailed accounts of his exciting adventures in dreamland.

One night when he realized that he was dreaming, Saint-Denys found himself at the top of a building. He noticed an open window and the pavement far below. "I plunged myself into the deep, curious and anxious at the same time."[19] When Saint-Denys awoke, he recalled a later scene in which people gathered around a dead man in a square in front of a cathedral. The man had jumped from the church tower, and Saint-Denys had watched the dead man be carried away on a stretcher. "This is the technique by which my memory and imagination had bypassed the trap set by me," he wrote in *Les*

Rêves. "With this familiarity I was in a dream quite often capable to repeat throwing myself off a high building or jumping into an abyss or deep well."[20]

In the late 1800s, a researcher at a women's liberal arts college was conducting dream experiments that would lead to one of today's most prominent concepts on dreaming. In 1890, Mary Whiton Calkins devised a novel dream experiment to explore the content of everyday dreams. For eight weeks, twenty-eight-year-old Calkins and her mentor, professor Edmund Sanford, recorded their dreams during the night. "For this purpose, paper, pencil, candle and matches were placed close at hand," wrote Calkins in "Statistics of Dreams," a research paper that recounted her experiment.

They collected dreams at different times, showing that sleep in the middle of the night is not in fact dreamless sleep. For the first few weeks, an alarm was used throughout the night. Yet it was soon discovered that waking to the shrill sound caused such excitement, it affected dream recall. Waiting until morning, though, ran the risk of forgetting the dream. One night, she woke to record her dream in the dark before she "sank off to sleep with the peaceful consciousness of a scientific duty well done." In the morning, she discovered that "an unsharpened pencil had been used, and the experimenter was left with a blank sheet of paper and no remotest memory of the dream, so carefully recalled after dreaming."[21] Reflecting on the dreams that escape our memory, she concluded that we dream much more than we might think.

Analyzing the collection of 375 dreams, Calkins discovered a close connection between our dreams and our waking lives, with only 11 percent of dreams lacking a connection between these states of consciousness.[22] Calkins' discovery of the "congruity and continuity" between our waking and dreaming lives lay the groundwork for psychologist Calvin Hall's Continuity Hypothesis, a 1970s model of dreaming that continues to be studied. Hall discovered that we don't simply dream about things that have happened during the day. We express our thoughts, preoccupations, and concerns in our dreams. The more we dream about someone or something, the more intense our concern is likely to be.

At the time, Calkins wasn't convinced of the importance of her findings.

In her 1930 autobiography, which was published thirty years after Freud's *The Interpretation of Dreams*, she characterized her conclusions on the dream-wake connection as "almost ludicrously opposed to the nowadays widely accepted Freudian conception of the dream; in fact, my study as a whole must be rather contemptuously set down by any good Freudian as superficially concerned with the mere 'manifest content' of the dream."[23]

Calkins made several other astute observations about the characteristics of a dream. She noted that the dreams occurred in the present. Even when the dreamer recalled their childhood home, they remained their actual age. Calkins observed that our most vivid dreams happen later in the night, which we now know is a characteristic of early morning REM dreams. Emotions expressed in dreams depend on the dreamer. What might be uncomfortable for some people may be enjoyable or pleasant for others. Calkins identified complex mental processes during dreaming, including imagination and real thought. She identified the normal and mundane aspects of dreaming. Calkins considered "the very prosaic and ordinary nature of most of the dreams recorded" to be the key finding of the experiment.[24]

Outside the laboratory at Wellesley College, Calkins continued to push boundaries. She taught philosophy at Boston College while she conducted her dream experiment. In order to teach a new course in the philosophy of the mind, Calkins needed to learn about psychology. As a favour to Wellesley College as well as to Calkins's father, a known Presbyterian minister, the president of Harvard University allowed Calkins to audit a psychology course. At the time, only men could attend Harvard.

Calkins was given a warm welcome by the men of the psychology department, including students and lab assistants. "I shall not let this opportunity pass by to record my gratitude for the friendly, comradely, and refreshingly matter-of-fact welcome," recalled Calkins in her autobiography.[25] During her time at Harvard, Calkins completed the requirements for a PhD in psychology. An unofficial defense for her dissertation was arranged by psychology faculty. Despite six professors recommending Calkins be awarded a doctorate, Harvard denied her a PhD because she was a woman. Yet Calkins felt "My debt, both academic and personal . . . must be acknowledged but can never be repaid."[26] A few years later, Radcliffe College, Harvard's sister college, offered Calkins a PhD. She refused the degree. During her forty years at Wellesley College, Calkins had an impressive career in research and teaching. She wrote several books, more than one hundred papers, and in 1905 was the first woman to become president of the American Psychological Association.

These early researchers shared a fascination with dreams, which guided their investigation of this mysterious other realm of existence. Throughout history, scholars, passionate dreamers, even royalty and rulers of ancient civilizations have studied the complex and confounding facets of dreams, from a fundamental understanding of what a dream is to its meaning, function, and possible use. In 2070 BC, the Egyptian Pharaoh Merikare's "dream book" described a dream as a looking glass into the future.[27] The ancient Egyptian language was a combination of words and symbols. The word for "dream" was *resut*, which translates as "awakening," and was paired with an open eye. Dreams were seen as a kind of purgatory between the living and the dead that could be visited by those on earth and those in the afterlife. Egyptians wrote "letters to the dead," asking favours from deceased family members and friends, and placed these in their tombs. In one letter, a sick man pleaded with his wife to meet him in a dream and ease his agony.[28]

There were the message dreams from 2000 BC in ancient Mesopotamia when everyone from kings to commoners saw their nightly stories as sources of guidance. In *The Epic of Gilgamesh*, the first recorded story written on clay tablets, King Gilgamesh, a tyrannical ruler famous for exerting his power on the battlefield and over his people, dreamt of a falling star that pinned him to the earth, rendering him defenseless. In the second century AD in Rome, the dream interpreter Artemidorus concluded that dreams could be reflections of our waking fears and desires or predictors of the future.

The Greek philosopher Aristotle saw a dream as a visual "presentation" of objects from our waking lives that we continue to think about during sleep. These images conjure new thoughts and emotions in our dreams. In Ancient China, dreams were revered as precious insights into the human psyche. During the fourth century BC, astrology was used to unearth the meaning of dreams.

For centuries, dreams have been understood as spiritual teachings. The Buddhist *Tibetan Book of the Dead* envisions death as ethereal and dream-like. If people can understand what it is to dream, their soul can rise above death as they pass away. The Bible describes dreams as celestial revelations. In Indigenous cultures around the world, dreams have always been sacred and of great value, sources of personal insight and a connection with our inner being.

Early dream researchers like Maury, Saint-Denys, and Calkins were confined to a psychological exploration of dreams. They relied on subjective reports that were filtered through the memory and perspective of the dreamer. With the advent of the EEG, the study of dreams took a radical turn. Dreaming could be examined as a physiological phenomenon. Then one night, an aspiring scientist from Brooklyn, New York, witnessed the sharp, staccato EEG lines of his son's dreaming brain, unravelling one of the great mysteries of the night.

Chapter Two

THE PEAKS AND
VALLEYS OF SLEEP

IN THE LATE 1940S, EUGENE ASERINSKY, A SLIM AND STRIKING
fellow from Brooklyn, New York, with blue eyes and jet-black hair, walked
into the physiology department of the University of Chicago in his characteristic black suit, ready to make his mark.

Life hadn't been easy for Aserinksy, who had lost his mother when he
was a boy and was raised by his often-absent Russian father. Boris Aserinsky
spent his days working as a dentist, but filling cavities wasn't how he made
his real money. When replacing an old filling, he would ask patients to discard the worn bit of metal down a spittoon, which had a built-in filter. He
would pry apart the spittoon to retrieve sparkling nuggets of silver and gold.
Every few weeks, Boris made the trek across the Brooklyn Bridge to visit the
precious metal dealers of Manhattan, who would weigh the silver and gold,
often paying him more than he'd earned for filling the cavities. Boris taught
his son the tricks of another one of his trades: gambling. At ten years old, he
spent many evenings playing four-handed pinochle, colluding with his dad
in front of unsuspecting players. The boy learned his dad's card signals. If it
was spades, he might scratch his right earlobe.[1]

When he arrived at the University of Chicago in his late twenties, Aserinsky possessed wisdom beyond his years. Accepted as a PhD candidate,
Aserinsky needed an advisor for his doctorate. He wasn't particularly inter-

ested in sleep. He simply wanted to study physiology. Yet he was struck by the credentials of Nathaniel Kleitman, known as the father of contemporary sleep research, who created the world's first sleep laboratory. Kleitman was renowned for his work in circadian rhythms and sleep deprivation. The American sleep researcher and physiologist had once stayed awake for 180 hours to study the effects of sleeplessness. In the late 1930s, Kleitman lived in Kentucky's Mammoth Cave for a month to observe the body's natural sleep-wake cycle. The fledgling student studied under Kleitman, an association that would become one of the most significant in the history of sleep medicine.

For an early assignment, Aserinsky stayed up all night, studying the blinking rate of infants to determine if it could be used to identify sleep onset, those first few minutes of sleep when we drift off. Kleitman had Aserinsky peer over the babies' cribs, studying their blinking as they nodded off. After many months, there wasn't much to report. Aserinsky noticed that the infants had wild eye movements after sleep onset, which seemed to stop suddenly during the night. At first, the exhausted student had taken advantage of these quiet periods, sneaking in much-needed naps before the infants awoke. But he started to wonder whether this activity had a reason or pattern.

It was the early 1950s, and researchers weren't yet collecting an entire night's recording of a patient's brain waves, the electrical impulses produced by the brain's nerve cells, or neurons. Years earlier in 1924, German psychiatrist Hans Berger had recorded the first electrical brain signals of a patient. Berger developed the electroencephalogram (EEG), offering a non-invasive method to study electrical brain activity. The brain test measures and records brain waves through electrodes that are placed on different areas of the skull.

Alpha waves appear when we're in a relaxed state of awareness, say if we're daydreaming or meditating. If you were to look at an expanded view of the waveforms, alpha waves look like rolling waves with rounded peaks and valleys. Beta waves arise when our thoughts are focused on something, say if we are trying to remember someone's name or we are engrossed in a conversation. In this wider view, they appear as tight, jagged scribbles. Theta waves may indicate we're in a state of deep relaxation, say if we're doing a mundane or routine task and we focus inwards, no longer noticing what we're doing. Theta waves also appear during light sleep in Stages 1 and 2. They look like ripples in the surface with the occasional rise or dip. Delta waves are associated with deep sleep. At this point, we're unaware of what's happening around us. The ripples become larger and lengthen, with the occasional hill or gentle slope.

In Aserinsky's time, it was known that sleep and wakefulness produce different brain activity. Yet many thought that during sleep, the brain switched off for a much-needed rest. If wakefulness was like water, sleep was like ice, thought Kleitman.[2] While Aserinsky spent most of his nights in the lab, his wife struggled at home. At four feet, ten inches, Sylvia was a "little slip of a person," said Aserinky's son Armond when I spoke with him many years ago. But she had always been a "sturdy soul," he explained. At home with two young children, Sylvia felt isolated and began to lose her characteristic strength and resilience. Armond, then nine, helped as much as he could, boiling bottles, making formula, and taking care of his baby sister. Sylvia's depression became her undoing, from which she never really recovered, said Armond. Aserinsky was a full-time student earning little or no money, and the family was barely surviving. He was determined to earn his PhD and secure a job.

Aserinsky found an old, abandoned EEG in the basement of the physiology building. He dragged the machine to a storage area with an adjoining room and set up a makeshift sleep lab with an army-style cot. This would allow him to sit in the adjoining room, monitoring his subject's eye movements, and brain waves on the EEG. All he needed was a patient, and his son volunteered. I asked Armond what the experience was like. "I wasn't reading this in the Hardy Boys, let me tell you. This was my own adventure," said Armond, who was fascinated by electronics as a kid. "This was fancy stuff. Uncharted territory."

At home, Aserinsky sometimes watched his son sleep, waking him to ask what was going through his mind. The boy would give his dad a play-by-play of his dreams. Armond slept over in the lab for two nights. He told me about being prepped for the sleep studies. First, he was rubbed almost raw with acetone at different spots along his face and head. Then his father gooped some paste onto various spots on his head and temples, placing the electrodes over the sticky substance, which itched when it dried. Tape was plastered across the electrodes to prevent them from moving. The colorful wires were attached loosely to Armond in case he rolled over in the night. These electrodes were wired to pens on the EEG that would transform the electrical signals from the brain into a topographical profile of rolling hills, low valleys, and sharp peaks across a landscape of blank paper.

During his first night in the lab, the young boy found it difficult to fall asleep. But soon exhaustion took hold, and he drifted off. A while later, Armond's eye movements scribbled wildly across the EEG. Aserinsky raced into the room to find Armond sound asleep, with his eyes darting back and forth under closed lids. The record seemed to indicate that the boy's brain was wide awake, even though he was clearly sleeping. At first, Aserinsky wondered if the EEG was playing tricks. Aserinsky made sure the machine was working properly, and Armond spent a second night in the lab. Aserinsky witnessed the same results. Armond was asleep while his brain churned with activity.

Aserinsky tested adults in the lab, observing that these peaked mountain ranges appeared on sleep records four or five times a night, with the associated eye movements. The young scientist discovered that heart rate and respiration rose during periods of high activity. Aserinsky started waking his subjects when their eyes darted back and forth, and they recounted vivid, bizarre dreams. But if he woke them when there was no sign of eye movements, they had hardly anything to report. It was difficult, though, to pick up REM sleep during every overnight study. In some cases, periods of REM were missed. "It was like hearing a voice on the radio saying, this is Mars calling, but you can't get it every night because there's static," explained Armond.

After conducting more than fifty sleep studies on two dozen subjects over the course of several months, Aserinsky assured himself that his results were not only accurate but of great importance. Armond recalled his father being so excited that he seemed almost agitated. When Aserinsky's research took this thrilling turn, Kleitman enlisted another student to help with the sleep studies.

In the fall of 1952, a University of Chicago medical student was intent on studying the unconscious mind in order to understand consciousness. Unlike Aserinsky, who focused on a scientific approach to dreaming, William Dement was fascinated by psychoanalysis. Listening to Aserinsky describe his findings, Dement was excited by the prospect of studying the mysterious dimension of dreams. When Dement heard that eye movements might be associated with dreaming, it was more stunning than being given a winning lottery ticket.[3] At the time, many thought that the brain shut down during sleep. It seemed impossible that the brain could generate eye movements similar to those of wakefulness.

Yet this is exactly what Dement and Aserinsky found. Using Kleitman's camera, the pair recorded 16-millimetre footage of patients in REM sleep. Until this point, researchers had conducted studies only on men, but Dement felt they should also study the sleep patterns of women. Kleitman didn't include women in overnight studies as he worried it would cause a scandal. The sleep doctor agreed to let Dement observe his girlfriend with Aserinsky present.[4] These observations along with other studies including women subjects showed that women experience REM sleep.

In the September 4, 1953, issue of *Science*, Aserinsky and Kleitman published their path-breaking study on rapid eye movement, propelling the field of sleep medicine. They showed that during REM, the brain is as active as when we are awake. This unbelievable REM activity happens every ninety minutes throughout the night. REM's discovery made headlines in *Time*, *The New York Times*, and *Newsweek* as scientists opened their eyes to the newfound world of sleep medicine.

Shortly after the groundbreaking discovery, Aserinsky left the field of sleep. He had earned his PhD, and in desperate need of a job, he took the first one offered and went to study salmon at Seattle's Bureau of Fisheries. Within a year, he began teaching physiology at Jefferson Medical College, where he stayed for more than two decades. Moving to Philadelphia brought his wife closer to her family. Yet nothing seemed to ease her depression. "She was ground down to dust," said Armond. At thirty-four years old, she died by suicide. Armond was fourteen.

Around the same time, Dement and Kleitman continued their quest to explore the uncharted world of sleep. They understood that sleep is not an idle state, and that REM whirs the brain into action several times a night. Dement and Kleitman contextualized REM within the sleep cycle. They discovered that we pass through a series of stages in our sleep and created a kind of traveller's guide for scientists to explore the bumpy roads, peaks, and valleys of the voyage. Their charting of the sleep cycle catapulted the field of sleep research to prominence, and scientists in other labs set off on their own explorations of the night. In 1970, Dement opened one of the first sleep disorders clinics at Stanford University to perform overnight sleep testing.

With these insights into the sleeping brain, researchers could look at dreams physiologically as well as psychologically to investigate what constitutes a dream. How does the brain create this common physiological phenomenon that is at the same time a personal psychological experience? As I turned this question over in my mind, I was reminded of a dream that I had when I was deep into the research for this book. I was spending a lot of time thinking about how to define a dream. I carried this seemingly simple yet confounding question with me into the night.

The Sleeping Brain

IT WAS THE END of March in Toronto, and after a stretch of warm weather that had convinced me to put away my winter boots, I sat at my desk, watching the snow fall. The heavy flakes were coming down fast, blanketing the tips of iris leaves and the vibrant yellow flowers of the forsythia tree that had bloomed unexpectedly the previous week. The snow softened the usual sounds of the school dismissal bell, my neighbour's car alarm, and a dump truck crashing over the speed bump in front of my house. My breathing slowed as I focused on the falling snowflakes and turned the increasingly puzzling question over again in my mind: What is a dream?

I had sifted through decades of dream research and interviewed many experts in the field. Yet I struggled to answer this fundamental question. The more I learned, the less I seemed to know. Every new insight raised a new question to explore. There were so many caveats and considerations that prevented me from landing on a definitive understanding of dreams.

When I drifted off and one thought dominoed into the next, did this constitute a dream? What about when my thoughts transformed into images? Or when these images took on a three-dimensionality and became my own home movie? How could a dream be something unexpected, even though I was the one who had created it? Is a dream a mental junkyard of random, disjointed ideas, a reflection of our biggest worries and preoccupations, or a combination of the mundane and the meaningful?

With these possibilities swirling around my mind, I looked down at small scraps of paper scattered across my desk. When an idea pops into my head, I find a piece of paper and scribble down the thought, even though I've got a pile of blank notebooks to organize my ideas. I enjoy working on several projects at once, which leads to a desk cluttered with possible ideas to chase.

Sitting at my desk, I stacked the pieces of paper and started shuffling through them. Some I could easily grasp while others escaped my memory or understanding. Did I write these? What had I been thinking? This made me think of how dreams are formed from a seemingly random collection of remembered thoughts, experiences, and emotions. Sometimes it's obvious how our dream thoughts reflect our waking lives while other times they appear illegible when we try to decode them. Even though we are the writers of our dreams, they can seem new and unpredictable. How, I wondered, does the brain construct a dream? What is happening inside the brain to generate a universal dream experience while creating nightly fictions that are uniquely our own?

That night, as the snowplows cleared the street in front of my house, I kept asking myself, what is a dream? I tossed and turned with the question. I flipped my pillow, rolled onto my side, and pressed my cheek into the cold cotton. A few hours earlier, my daughter had played "Style" by Taylor Swift while we were making dinner. The song played on an endless loop in my head. Gradually, the lyrics turned into images. I imagined red lipsticked lips. Headlights following the curves of a country road that I drove as a teenager. The laughing face of an old friend. I fell asleep with the ripped pieces of paper swirling around my head.

IN MY DREAM, I am hunched over my desk, determined to glue the pieces of paper together, but their jagged edges make it impossible. I catch sight of a spool of thread dancing through the air. I watch the thread slip through the eye of a needle. The bits of paper become colourful squares, and the floating needle sews them into a quilt. I sit back from my desk and enjoy a cathartic sigh. Then suddenly, someone snips the thread and the squares float into the air like helium-filled balloons. I try to catch them and grab fistfuls of air as the tiny pieces of paper remain just out of reach. Eventually, they drift away into an endless blue sky.

Jump cut to a new scene. I'm dragging a purple bag down a quiet suburban street. I realize it's the town where I grew up. I see that I'm holding someone's hand. I look up and find my mother walking beside me. The bag is so heavy it's making my arm grow longer as I pull it along with us. I stop walking to eat a bunch of purple grapes.

Without warning, I find myself in the small library where I spent countless hours as a kid. There are orange upholstered benches and a rainbow of colourful, round carpets set up for story time. I stand in front of the card catalogue and open a long, thin wooden drawer. Instead of finding index cards with call numbers for each book, there are translucent boxes housing my scraps of paper. I pull the drawer toward me and find dozens of clear boxes. I remove one of the boxes and try to pry it open, but it's stuck. After a lot of effort, the box bursts open and instead of a piece of paper, one of my dreams floats through the air. I watch the dream scene play out as it drifts through a vast blue sky that has replaced the library's speckled foam tiled ceiling. I start opening the drawers of the card catalogue to reveal box after translucent box of dreams. Somehow, I know that all the dreams I've ever had are within these wooden drawers.

I pop open another clear box and find that it's one of my favourite dreams. I wish I could tell you what it is. All I know is that I'm excited to see it again. It's snowing now, and the dream starts to drift away. As I lunge for it, I am transported back to my office. Sitting at my desk, I look out the window at the falling snow. I glance down to find the letters erased from my keyboard. I tell myself that I don't need to see the letters to type; that everything will be OK. Then my office fills with smoke. There's the shrill, monotone beep of a smoke alarm. I bolt awake to find that it's the sound of my alarm. I grab the paper and pen on my bedside table and scribble down what I can remember of the dream while the last scene floats through my mind.

How did my brain create this dream? As I delved into the workings of the sleeping brain, I discovered that brain activity is different in non-REM (NREM) and REM sleep. There are three NREM sleep stages and one final stage of REM sleep. We travel through the sleep cycle several times a night, moving in and out of NREM and REM sleep.

The Sleep Cycle

IMAGINE SETTLING INTO YOUR bed at the end of a long day. With eyes closed, your mind sifts through thoughts and experiences. Maybe you are reliving certain moments or, if you are like me, writing mental to-do lists for the next day. At this point, you are still aware of the world around you. The mattress might feel hard and unforgiving as you toss and turn, looking for a comfortable position. Maybe you notice the booming bass from a passing car or recognize sounds from another room.

You forget about your surroundings as your mind drifts from one thought to the next, transforming into images, often plucked from earlier in the day, that are replaced as fast as you can imagine them. This is sleep onset, when you cross the bridge between wakefulness and sleep. Sleep onset moves from wakefulness to drowsiness to sleep.

During the first few minutes of sleep, the things we choose to think about might not be as accidental or disconnected as they seem. In several studies, Robert Stickgold found that during sleep onset, our brain tags important memories to revisit later during sleep. What makes memories important to us? We will explore this in chapter six when we investigate the relationship between memory and sleep.

The light and airy Stage 1 of the sleep cycle lasts only a few minutes. Your muscles relax, and you might have the occasional twitch. Sleep onset includes Stage 1. Imagine the sleep onset process as a sandwich, explained dream researcher Adam Haar. One piece of bread is wakefulness and the other piece is Stage 2. Stage 1 is in between the two slices.

From Stage 1, you drift quickly into Stage 2. This is when your breathing, heart rate, and brain waves slow, punctuated by quick bursts of brain activity, known as sleep spindles. Stage 2 lasts ten to twenty-five minutes in your first round of the sleep cycle and gets longer as you repeat the cycle throughout the night.

Stage 3, also called slow-wave sleep or deep sleep, is characterized by large, rolling brain waves known as delta waves. It is the deepest stage of NREM and the hardest to wake up from. Some people won't even notice music blaring if they're in deep sleep. If you wake up during this stage, it can take a while for the mental fog to clear. Sleepwalking often happens during Stage 3. Deep sleep helps the body repair itself and bolster the immune system. NREM occurs across Stages 1 to 3. About three quarters of the time we spend asleep is in NREM.

The final stage of the sleep cycle is REM. It was named "paradoxical sleep" by French neurophysiologist Michel Jouvet to reflect REM's contradictory nature in which the body is paralyzed while the mind is as active as when you are awake. During REM, your brain hums with activity, your heart rate and respiration increase, and your eyes, although shut, typically dart back and forth in a continual staccato as if you were reading a book.

The first REM period happens around ninety minutes after you fall asleep. Periods of REM become longer as the night progresses. We repeat the sleep cycle around four to five times a night, moving in and out of NREM and REM sleep. While we dream throughout the night, our more bizarre, emotional, and vivid dreams tend to happen in REM sleep, which has distinct brain activity compared to NREM sleep.

During NREM sleep, brain activity slows down. Then when we move from NREM into REM sleep, activity increases in different areas of the brain. The brain's limbic centre, which helps process and regulate emotions, and the medial prefrontal cortex, which plays a role in autobiographical memory and emotions, become more active. At the same time, activity in much of the prefrontal cortex, which helps us make decisions, control impulses, and think rationally, quiets down during REM sleep compared to when we're awake. Think of those vivid, bizarre dreams in which you seem to go along with the strange series of events. During REM sleep, the neurotransmitters GABA (gamma-aminobutyric acid) and glycine work together to suppress activity of motor neurons in the spinal cord, which paralyzes our muscles and prevents us from acting out our dreams. This brain mechanism is faulty in people with REM behaviour disorder, letting them act out their dreams, which can be terrifying or dangerous, causing the dreamer to punch, scream, or jump out of bed.

The combination of brain activity allows us to navigate our dream worlds and experience emotions and sensations that simulate waking life. When we dream, we are disconnected from the outside world. We aren't processing external information around us. So the dreaming brain taps into memories to generate content. Later in the book, we will explore how the brain decides which memories are dream-worthy.

There are many facets to a dream. It is a universal physiological phenomenon that can be explained through brain activity. It is also a psychological experience that is personal and unique to each of us. This raises the question that has inspired and mystified dream researchers since they set their sights on the world of dreams: What is the meaning of dreams? Are they meaningful in and of themselves, or does our waking mind assign meaning based on our unique combination of associations, knowledge, and perspectives? Could dreams be meaningless by-products of sleep? Do we dismiss our dreams or mine them for meaning, sifting through the mundane and bizarre details to find precious insights and shimmers of creativity? Or is there a more nuanced approach to the debate?

When I reflected on my dream of a dream, I thought about how it pushed me to think differently about dreaming, how every night we search our mental catalogue of memories and piece together stories to experience and possibly remember. It shone a spotlight on some thoughts and feelings that I wasn't paying attention to. Most of all, my dream let me revisit forgotten moments that now seem quite special in their own quiet, unassuming way.

Take a moment and think back to a dream that has stuck with you. Maybe it's a terrifying one that you can't shake or maybe it's so cryptic that you are compelled to share and try to decode it. What could it mean? This brings us back to Freud, who is forever at the centre of this debate, and the work of two sleep and dream scientists on opposite sides of the father of dreams.

Cryptograms of the Mind

AS A BOY, J. Allan Hobson spent countless hours performing experiments in the cellar of his childhood home in Hartford, Connecticut. With his father's help, Hobson put up walls and built benches for his very own chemistry lab. The boy would cut open snakes and watch their insides continue to writhe about, trying to understand how the body is connected to the brain. A woman who helped around the house told Hobson that the snake's insides would slither around only until sundown, but he was doubtful. Trying the experiment at night, Hobson found that everything moved just as it did during the day.

"I began, I think, to realize that most of what people told you was unsubstantiated. They were just beliefs," the late Hobson explained during one of our long chats some years ago. "It was folk psychology and folk religion, and I developed a deeply skeptical attitude, which was extremely helpful in science." To be a good scientist, "you have to realize that most of what you think about the true nature of reality is an illusion."

We spoke for several hours, exploring the many facets of dreaming. We discussed everything from the father of dreams ("Freud is a genius," he said. "The only problem is, he just made things up.") to the similarities between our dreams, despite our different histories and the myths we created about ourselves. "We're probably both capable of being crazy, in the daytime as well as the nighttime sense of the word," he explained. "All we need is some sort of a loss in our lives or some trauma. I think the whole thing is up for grabs." We talked about the importance of treating subjective experience as data in dream research, with so much to learn from the alternate realm of dream experience. Through his own story, Hobson highlighted the importance of curiosity and skepticism to push the bounds of thinking and possibility.

Hobson told me of his dad's profound influence on his life. His father was a patent attorney with a passion for engineering as well as naturalism. His dad loved the outdoors and spent a lot of time in the woods near their home. He had many inventor friends who were often around, immersing Hobson in their fascinating discoveries. "Who you meet is who you become," said Hobson as he explained their influence during his early life. "They were trying to design new ways of doing things, and that's what science is all about," he said.

Hobson attended Harvard Medical School, where he studied neuroscience and psychiatry. Yet he was frustrated by the lack of objective scientific study. "If you were trying to be a psychiatrist, you had to know what all of your historical hang-ups were," he said. "It was ridiculous. So insulting." Then Fred Snyder at the National Institutes of Health told Hobson he could actually tell, just by looking at a sleep record, when patients were dreaming. Hobson remembers the moment he saw the unbelievably active waves of the sleeping brain. "That night was like a religious experience," he said. "There was an objective basis for some sort of correlation between the brain and the mind."[5] Once he caught a glimpse of those brain waves, the young scientist set out to investigate the complexities of the sleeping brain. "I decided that I really wouldn't be happy standing outside the brain. I needed to be inside."

Hobson spent some time in France working with Michel Jouvet, the French neuroscientist who had shown that neurons fire spontaneously while we are asleep, including neurons in the brain stem that play a pivotal part in generating REM sleep. Jouvet discovered during a series of experiments with cats how the body is paralyzed during REM sleep while the mind buzzes with activity.[6]

Jouvet's sleep studies came about quite by accident. He was examining the brain of cats to understand the process of learning. However, his cats weren't as enthusiastic. Jouvet tried to get them to learn a new task, but the animals kept falling asleep. When they slipped into REM, Jouvet noticed that they lay there, paralyzed. Jouvet then cut specific nerves to stop the usual muscle paralysis during REM. When the cats drifted into REM sleep, they would start sleepwalking, crawling around as if on an imaginary prowl.

Jouvet hooked up his cats to an EEG machine to compare brain activity during sleep and waking when they learned something new. He discovered that the cats' EEG recordings became activated during REM just like when they were awake. His cats were asleep. They had lost their ability to move. Yet their brains remained awake. Reflecting on this irony, Jouvet referred to REM as "paradoxical sleep." In another experiment, Jouvet discovered that the pons area in the brain stem plays a pivotal role in generating and regulating REM sleep. But how? Hobson imagined there was a kind of clock ticking away inside the brain stem that turned REM on and off, and he was determined to find it.

In the late sixties, Hobson set up a sleep lab at the Massachusetts Mental Health Center to study the sleeping brain. At the time, Robert McCarley was a psychiatry resident. He shared Hobson's enthusiasm and joined the lab. The pair continued to investigate what was happening in the brain stem during REM. "Everybody thought the brain was going to turn off during sleep," said Hobson. "They were all wrong."

Then in 1977, Hobson and McCarley put forth the activation-synthesis model of dreaming. It proposed that the pons area of the brain stem is activated during dreaming and produces partly random information. This process also activates stored memories. Then the activated forebrain tries to piece together, or *synthesize*, the information with other stored memories, creating a dream. "In other words, the forebrain may be making the best of a bad job in producing even partially coherent dream imagery from the relatively noisy signals sent up to it from the brain stem," wrote Hobson and McCarley in their influential paper in the *American Journal of Psychiatry*.[7]

The paper called into question psychoanalytic dream theory. "The primary motivating force for dreaming is not psychological but physiological since the time of occurrence and duration of dreaming sleep are quite constant, suggesting a preprogrammed, neurally determined genesis."[8] Yet there were nuances to the argument. Hobson and McCarley contended that their new theory did not in fact deny possible meaning of dreams. Instead, it proposed a "more direct route to their acquisition" through physiological processes instead of free association and the disguised wishes suggested by Freud. They believed that dreams are driven by neuronal firings of the brain stem, not psychological motivation or repression.

In the years leading up to Hobson and McCarley's pivotal work, dreams were rarely reported outside of REM sleep. Yet when subjects were woken during REM, they reported dreams most of the time. Psychologist David Foulkes decided to waken patients before their EEG patterns signalled REM sleep to see what was happening. Foulkes had some startling results when he asked what was on people's minds rather than if they were dreaming. More than half of the reports showed that people were "dreaming" outside of REM. Foulkes discovered that dreams during NREM sleep could be complex and emotional like dreams during REM. Although these tend to happen during longer, later periods of NREM.[9]

Were dreaming and REM sleep their own separate states, generated by different brain activity? Scientists continued to investigate the brain mechanisms of dreaming. Then along came a curious graduate student in South Africa intent on bridging the brain-mind divide who, in the process, called into question why we dream.

Rewriting Freud's Obituary

IT COULD BE SAID that Mark Solms's study of the mind began when he was just four years old and witnessed a tragic accident that would change the course of his brother's life. It was the 1960s, and the Solms family was living in a small village in Namibia. They had decided to spend a warm afternoon at their yacht club. While their parents went out on the water, Solms and his six-year-old brother, Lee, stayed back at the clubhouse to play with other children.

The group of boys raced around the club while Solms tried to keep up. Some of the bigger boys decided to climb up the back of the clubhouse that was built on a ridge. It was too far a climb for Solms, who watched his older brother from the pavement below. Running around on the roof with the other boys, Lee raced to the front, then suddenly lost his balance. Solms watched his brother fall nearly twenty feet to the pavement below. Then came the whirring of a helicopter that transported Lee to Cape Town for emergency brain surgery.

When Lee returned home six weeks later, he was very different, explained Solms during one of our conversations. Their imaginary games no longer interested Lee. Pretending to dig for diamonds in their make-believe mine or playing battlefield in the sand now seemed ridiculous to him. When Solms built a castle out of Lego, Lee would smash it apart. When they played war, Solms would devise a set of elaborate rules to follow, while Lee simply wanted them to hit each other. It was a confusing experience for the young Solms. The boy thought, This is not my brother. This is some other person. "But clearly, he is my brother because he looks the same. He's got the same name," said Solms when he explained his thinking at the time. "The question really was, Where is my real brother? Where has he gone?" Solms felt like he had lost his one true friend and playmate. At such a young age, Solms didn't understand how brain damage could change a person.

When it was time to go to university, Solms decided to study the brain. It was 1980, and the field focused on processing and cognitive capacity. Solms was fascinated by neuropsychology. At the time, he didn't connect his chosen field with his brother. "Without me realizing it, I was looking for something much more hard to find," he said. "Answers to these great mysteries of how we are our brains. How a bodily organ can somehow be your very self, your being, your existence." Solms was advised to avoid such metaphysical topics. He became increasingly frustrated and disappointed when professors suggested he focus on more scientific questions.

"How can it be that a person like my brother can be lost because his brain has been damaged? The whole person changes. The whole being changes," said Solms. "What was left out of neuroscience was the thing that I must have been so forcibly confronted with as a child, which was, the brain is the person, the brain is the self, the brain is who you are."

In addition to the "cerebral problem-solving detective work of diagnosis," Solms discovered that he had a deep need to help people with brain disease. "You know, for the obvious reason that they were people like my brother," said the psychoanalyst and neuropsychologist who coincidentally now works in the Cape Town hospital where his brother had brain surgery.

During one of our calls, Solms took me back to 1984 when he read *A Leg to Stand On* by Oliver Sacks. Solms recited a line that has stayed with him over all these years. "Neuropsychology is admirable, but it excludes the psyche—it excludes the experiencing, active, living 'I,'" wrote Sacks.[10] Solms found it remarkable that while psychology studied the mind, neuropsychology studied objective mechanisms and left the mind out of the picture. Solms wrote to Sacks and began a lifelong friendship with the British author and neurologist.

For his doctoral research, Solms focused on the brain mechanisms of dreaming. In the 1980s, the aspect of consciousness that was a respectable research topic in neuropsychology was sleep and waking. The remarkable thing about dreams, noted Solms, was that we become conscious while we are asleep. His professors focused on the study of sleep. Yet Solms was interested in dreaming. So he enrolled in a Freud seminar in the humanities department and learned about Freudian dream theory as well as Freud's background in neuroscience. He read Freud's "Project for a Scientific Psychology" and began to realize that "this field of psychoanalysis, for all its faults—and my God, it has big faults, too," he told me, "but at least it takes seriously the lived life of the mind as its subject matter." Psychoanalysis studied the mind in the full sense, examining thoughts and emotions rather than just the brain's physiology.

Freud was fascinated by depth psychology and the study of the unconscious. Solms aimed to bridge psychoanalysis and neuroscience to create a comprehensive understanding of the brain within the person, something impossible in Freud's day without advances in brain science.

In 1988, at the age of twenty-seven, Solms moved to London to train in psychoanalysis and work simultaneously in the neurosurgery department of the Royal London Hospital. For a neuroscientist to train in psychoanalysis was like admitting he had a sideline as a palm reader. Working in both fields, Solms quickly discovered that while neuroscience needed the theoretical concepts of psychoanalysis, psychoanalysis required the research methods of neuroscience to make its theories more evidence-based and experimentally tested.

To piece together how different parts of the brain are involved in the dreaming process, Solms studied the effects on dreaming of damage to certain brain regions. He found that patients with lesions in the pons area of the brain stem had a loss of REM sleep. This made sense, considering the pons is crucial for generating REM sleep. Surprisingly, these patients continued to dream. One after another, patients reported vivid dreams despite the loss of REM sleep. Could this mean that REM and dreaming were controlled by separate brain processes? Then Solms discovered patients with lesions in their forebrain didn't report any dreams. Yet they continued to have REM sleep. It was an absolutely fortuitous and accidental discovery.

Solms found a group of patients with damage to one precise part of the frontal lobes on both sides simultaneously, which was extremely rare. Solms explained that there are few diseases that produce these lesions in the exact same spot on both sides of the frontal lobes. It was a stroke of luck that among his 360 patients, Solms discovered nine people who had this exact type of damage in the deep frontal white matter of the brain. None of the patients reported dreams. Yet they continued to have REM sleep. Solms had another striking observation. He discovered that these nine patients lacked motivation. They were inert and apathetic, he explained.

Solms sifted through past scientific literature and discovered that patients who had frontal leucotomies, a psychosurgery to reduce hallucinations and delusions, also reported a loss of dreaming. This operation cut the same fibres in the brain that were damaged in Solms's group of nine patients who had stopped reporting their dreams. Solms read a paper by a German psychosurgeon that stated if a patient continued to dream after a leucotomy, the operation was deemed a failure because of the close association between dreams and psychosis. "That's what dreaming is," Solms told me. "It's a hallucinatory, delusional state of mind." Solms discovered further evidence that dreaming is not synonymous with REM sleep. He noted that more than forty-four patients with lesions in the forebrain didn't report dreams while they continued to have REM sleep. In addition, eighteen patients with lesions in the brainstem didn't have REM sleep but continued to experience dreams.[11] The question then became, what is so critical in the forebrain for generating hallucinations and delusions? If this mechanism could be identified, it might help to explain what causes dreams.

In the 1950s, antipsychotic medications offered a non-invasive, reversible treatment to replace the frontal leucotomy. The way these meds work is by blocking dopamine transmission in the brain. Dopamine is the brain chemical behind our reward system, also known as our wanting system. It provides positive motivation. If we participate in something thrilling or pleasurable, we get a surge of dopamine. By blocking dopamine, these medications were able to stop the hallucinations associated with psychiatric disorders like schizophrenia. Blocking dopamine also affected dreaming. Solms reflected on his nine patients who did not report any dreams and at the same time lacked motivation.

Solms then discovered another group of patients with brain damage in the basal forebrain (in the transitional zone between the brain stem and the forebrain). Rather than being unable to dream, the patients dreamt all the time. When they were awake, they were bombarded with hallucinations. If they thought about a person, they might actually see a hallucination of the person standing in front of them.

Solms referred to functional neuroimaging studies that showed that certain forebrain mechanisms are involved in the dreaming process, and that our dreams are made using complex cognitive processes. Solms pointed out that dreams involve our emotional forebrain. While the civilized, rational, intellectual parts of the brain shut down during dreams, the brain's emotional centre is active. "The part of the brain that generates our interest, our motivation, our volition, our intentionality is the part of the brain that generates our dreams," said Solms. "Therefore, there is every reason to believe that dreams are those things. They are intentional, motivated, meaningful states of volition."

Mentioning Freud's name "is like a red rag to a bull," said Solms. While it is clear that some of Freud's ideas were wrong, it's an injustice to science to dismiss his work entirely. In dreams, we have access to parts of ourselves that often remain under the surface of our awareness. "I think that dreams reveal something about what matters to us," said Solms. If we study someone's dreams, we learn something about what is important to them and what they care about.

"I never said that dreams were meaningless. I never said they were entirely nonsensical," said Hobson, who kept track of his own dreams, filling more than one hundred volumes. "There is a chaotic, nonsensical aspect to it. The reason for that is the brain is activated in a different way." The brain operates without the same participation of the prefrontal cortex. "The problem people have is they are sure that these [dreams] are cryptograms of their mind," said Hobson. The unconscious isn't a repository of negative and unacceptable material, as Freud attested. There is a transparency to dreams, which lets people examine them at face value.

More recently, Hobson and British neuroscientist Karl J. Friston proposed a new theory of dreams that suggested REM sleep plays a pivotal role in updating our mental reconstructions of the world. When we are awake, we interact with others and our environment to create a virtual model of the world. Our brains update this model constantly with new experiences and ideas. In dreams, events seem as real to us as waking experiences. The neuroscientists proposed that dreams, specifically during REM sleep, create a simulated reality that help us refine and optimize our reconstructions of the waking world and ourselves.[12] In this way, our dreaming brain goes offline to tweak our virtual model of the world. Then we come back online to waking consciousness with an updated model that helps to guide our thoughts and experiences.

In recent years, scientists have studied areas of the brain that are linked to dreaming as well as daydreaming. When we dream during REM sleep, we fire up the brain's default mode network (DMN), which is also associated with mind-wandering. The DMN involves several brain regions doing different things at the same time. Let's say I'm daydreaming about our family vacation to Italy a few years ago. While I'm reminiscing about the day we snorkeled and bobbed around the Mediterranean Sea, other areas of my brain remain aware of my surroundings, keeping me safe while I daydream.

We spend a third of our lives asleep, or trying to sleep, and a large portion of that time dreaming. A big part of our waking hours is spent daydreaming. Daydreaming and dreaming are both associated with the DMN. In fact, G. William Domhoff and Kieran Fox propose that dreaming, specifically during REM sleep, is an "intensified form of mind-wandering."[13] While they noted that dreams are longer and more visual and immersive than mind-wandering, both states of consciousness use some of the same brain regions in the DMN, with differing levels of activity.

As Hobson pointed out, subjective experience is data that is worthy of scientific study, and it is directly accessible. All we need is a paper and pen, and we can do all kinds of experiments from tracing memory sources to doing content analysis of how dreams depict waking life. By learning about the dreaming process and our perception and reactions in this altered state of consciousness, we are given new perspectives on ourselves. While not all dreams are meaningful, we might find glimmers of insight, especially when they echo preoccupations or worries from waking life.

At times, dreams go against people's wishes and intentions. Next on my tour through the world of dreams, I explored parasomnias, including a sleep disorder that compels people to act out their dreams, sometimes with disastrous consequences.

Chapter Three

THE DARK SIDE OF
THE DREAMING MIND

ONE WARM JULY EVENING IN 2003, JAN LUEDECKE ARRIVED AT A
house party in the Beaches, a leafy Toronto neighbourhood of dead-end
streets dotted with Victorian and Edwardian houses that lead to Lake
Ontario. It was the busiest time of year for the owner of a landscaping company. He was also tired from a cottage party the previous night, where he'd
drank and eaten some magic mushrooms—not to mention the four funerals
he'd attended recently. Yet it was his friend's annual croquet tournament.
Luedecke had won the previous year and was ready to defend his title.

A woman, known as L.O., arrived around the same time. There were
about fifty people at the party, drinking and playing croquet. Luedecke consumed around a dozen beers, a couple of rum and Cokes, and a couple of
vodkas. At around 2 a.m., L.O. curled up in the corner of a sectional couch.
While she waited for her friends to leave, she fell asleep in the living room. A
couple of hours later, Luedecke fell asleep on the opposite end of the couch.

L.O. awoke to find Luedecke on top of her. Taking in the situation, she
realized that this stranger was having sex with her. L.O. shoved Luedecke
to the floor. "Who are you, like what are you doing?" she demanded before
scooping up her things and racing for the door. A few minutes later, L.O
returned for her car keys to find Luedecke standing there, frozen, in the living room. Luedecke later said that he was in a state of shock. "This girl was

running around screaming at me and I didn't know what had happened."[1] When L.O. asked Luedecke his name, he answered. She didn't remember him from the party.

When she made her statement to the police, L.O. described Luedecke after she had pushed him off her. "He looked completely incoherent. Like not even when someone's drunk. More like just when you've just woken them up out of a sound sleep."[2]

After the incident, Luedecke went to his parents' house a few blocks away and fell back asleep. When he awoke and went to the bathroom, he discovered that he was wearing a condom. Luedecke flushed it down the toilet before padding back to bed. Later on, Luedecke called his friend who had hosted the party. The police were at his friend's house looking for a man who had allegedly committed sexual assault. Luedecke asked to talk to the police. He told the detective that he thought he was the perpetrator.

At the station, Luedecke tried to piece the night together. But it wasn't like trying to recall ordinary memories. He described his thoughts as hazy and vague, almost like a vision he watched from the outside.[3] Luedecke was arrested and charged with sexual assault.

When the case went to court in 2005, Luedecke pleaded not guilty with a defence of non-insane automatism. According to Luedecke's lawyers, when he had sex with L.O., he wasn't aware of what he was doing. Luedecke acted against his conscious will during sleep. How could he do this without recollection or intent? Luedecke's lawyers explained that he suffered from sexsomnia, also known as sleep sex, an erotic type of parasomnia.

Out of Touch

PARASOMNIAS ARE A KIND of sleep disorder characterized by a mixed brain state. Some parasomnias cause people to do activities they wouldn't normally do in their sleep like walk, talk, eat, or have sex. With parts of their brain awake while other areas of the brain are asleep, people have enough control to navigate the waking world and do complex tasks like drive or cook a meal, typically if they're in a familiar place. In the morning, people don't usually remember their actions, and they're left to piece together a story from clues or evidence from the previous night. People who sleep-walk might wake up in a strange place, while those who eat in their sleep might awaken surrounded by candy wrappers.

Parasomnias occur in NREM and REM sleep. Every night, we travel through the sleep cycle four to five times, dipping in and out of NREM and REM sleep. This nocturnal journey doesn't go so smoothly for people with a parasomnia. The rarest type of parasomnia occurs during REM sleep. REM behaviour disorder affects approximately 1 percent of the general population and about 2 percent of older adults. The prevalence is much higher among people with Parkinson's disease, at about 50 percent to 60 percent.[4] For most of us, our muscles are paralyzed during REM, which prevents us from acting out our dreams. We remain frozen except for our eyes, which typically dart back and forth, and our chests, which rise and fall with breath. But for those with REM behaviour disorder, the body is free to move, often with dangerous consequences. Some people have jumped out of windows to escape imagined attackers, while others fall down flights of stairs, breaking bones, or wake up with their hands around their partner's neck, convinced they are defending themselves. Carlos H. Schenck and Mark Mahowald of the Minnesota Regional Sleep Disorders Centre were the first to document human cases of REM behaviour disorder in the mid-1980s.

A more common parasomnia that occurs mostly during REM sleep is nightmare disorder. Nightmares are disturbing and sometimes trauma-related dreams that are often left unresolved as the person bolts awake to escape the terrifying situation. Approximately 5 percent of the general population have regular nightmares, with at least one per week, while many people have an occasional nightmare. Nightmares are more common among children, while women tend to have more nightmares than men.[5]

Night terrors are a different kind of parasomnia that affects about 2 percent to 4 percent of the population. They occur during Stage 3 deep sleep and cause a physical reaction. Some people scream out in terror, feel the wild thumping of their racing heart, or bolt awake in a panicked state of confusion.

Somnambulism, commonly known as sleepwalking, also occurs during deep sleep, when parts of the brain have lost touch with the waking world and the body isn't yet paralyzed by REM sleep. This is when people experience sudden "arousals." These mini-awakenings don't snatch the entire brain from sleep and reconnect it with the outside world. It's a mixed brain state of activity.

It's thought that sleepwalkers "for various reasons, have difficulties transitioning from slow-wave sleep to wakefulness. They get stuck in between," said sleep researcher Antonio Zadra. Across numerous studies on sleepwalking, Zadra and other dream researchers examined the EEGs of sleepwalkers and found that parts of the brain were still asleep. The subjects had high amplitude delta waves, which are found in Stage 3 deep sleep, while other areas of the brain were partially or fully awake. This may explain why sleepwalkers can navigate their environment. It may also account for some impaired judgement. "They can open doors and get dressed. They see things. They respond to them," said Zadra, adding, "They might misconstrue them." This can make people do strange things in their sleep.

Zadra offered the example of a sleepwalker who grabbed his dog that was asleep on the bed, put the dog in the tub, and turned on the shower. Why would he do such a thing? When the man opened his eyes during these episodes, he saw his dog, which was actually on the bed. But he also saw imaginary flames shooting off the dog, which he tried to douse with water. "You can get things superimposed, or you misinterpret what you see," said Zadra. He told me another example of a man who mistook a red power light in his room for the laser sight of a sharpshooter. Often, sleepwalkers are driven by a specific impulse or motivation, which can trigger a sense of urgency to act.

Why do people sleepwalk? One factor is genetics. Sleepwalking may run in families. If you suffer from a parasomnia as a child, there is a greater chance you will experience one later in life. There are certain triggers that can set off an episode in sleepwalkers. Exhaustion as well as alcohol can affect deep sleep, which increases the risk of parasomnias that happen during this sleep stage. Stress can be another contributing factor.

Sleepwalkers may appear awake, yet out of touch. Some grab their car keys and head for the road. Others crawl across the bed toward their partner to have drowsy sleep sex. If it's food that people crave, they might find their way to the kitchen, wielding knives and operating a hot stove to satisfy their real or imagined hunger. Sleep eating is a type of parasomnia that can devastate lives. People gorge themselves on gallons of ice cream and boxes of cereal. Some sleep eaters drink house paint and eat raw chicken. They wake up in the morning covered in vomit, develop ulcers and digestive disorders, and gain weight. In an interview with *The New York Times*, sleep and dream researcher Carlos H. Schenck explained that sleep eating might happen when our mind confuses the instinctual behaviours of sleeping and eating, and these instincts become intertwined.[6]

A Switch That Gets Stuck

TO LEARN MORE ABOUT sleep eating, possible triggers, and its effect on a person's life, I met with Janet Makinen, who for several years struggled with this parasomnia. She shared her story of sleep eating when I reached her in Florida many years ago.

Makinen's troubles began in the late 1990s when she awoke one morning around 4 a.m. to go to the bathroom. Padding down the hallway of her Tampa bungalow, she flicked on the bathroom light and was stunned by her surroundings. The sink and mirror were caked with soot and a box of Band-Aids had been left on the counter. She lowered her gaze and found a trail of black dust on the floor. Makinen followed the trail to the kitchen, turned on the light and was shaken by the scene before her. There were shards of burnt aluminum foil in the sink, a thin dusting of soot covered the counter and floor, and the inside of the microwave was blackened and burned. Milk was splattered across the floor. "It looked like a pack of teenagers had gone through my kitchen," Makinen told me. The only other person in the house was her husband, John.

Makinen stormed back down the hallway and burst into their bedroom to confront her husband. Then she eyed something puzzling on her side of the bed and fell silent. John awoke to his wife standing over him, and followed her gaze to the sheets, which were smeared with something brown. "That's blood," he exclaimed. Makinen looked at the substance carefully. That's not blood, she realized. That's barbecue sauce. What was he doing cooking in the middle of the night, she wanted to know. But John had been asleep. Panic swelled inside of her. Had they been broken into? Was there someone in the house at that very moment? They listened for an intruder. The house was silent.

When the couple went to the kitchen, they found the aftermath of a feast. Food was everywhere. John pointed to the burned microwave with bits of aluminum foil. Something on Makinen's hands caught her attention. Her fingers were covered in bandages. Taking in the scene, Makinen began to shake. "Oh my God," she said. "What's wrong with me?"

Makinen knew that she was stressed out. Things hadn't been easy lately. The couple had almost finished building their new house in Dade City when it was robbed, stripped of the kitchen appliances and Jacuzzi. At the same time, sleep troubles weren't new to Makinen. She had been an insomniac since she was a teenager. She told me how she would stay up for days until she began to hallucinate, seeing faces pass by her bedroom window. Even as a kid, Makinen didn't sleep much. Once her family had drifted off, she would slip out of the house to the barn, saddle up her horse, and go riding in the woods. Other times she climbed onto the roof with a blanket and lay beneath the stars. As an adult, she had spent many nights tossing and turning, unable to sleep.

In 1998, Makinen was prescribed Ambien (zolpidem) for her sleeplessness. The drug is fast-acting and causes most people to drift off within minutes. Its sedative effect is similar to a benzodiazepine like Valium in that it affects GABA, a neurotransmitter in the brain that sends messages between brain cells. GABA is like the brain's built-in hypnotist, commanding neurons to slow their staccato firing and take it easy for a while. Ambien targets GABA and helps to calm the whirring brain so people with insomnia can get some rest. For the first few weeks she was on the drug, Makinen had no problems. But then she began to eat, and eat, and eat. "If you're out in the desert for a while and you haven't had any water and you come upon a small body of water, you don't just drink a little bit," she told me. "You drink as much as your body can hold. It was like a survival flip in my head. It didn't matter what the food was. I was just shoving it in my mouth."

One morning she walked into the kitchen to find chips and candy strewn everywhere. The tops of cereal boxes had been ripped off, and a hot dog had been left on the counter. Makinen, who is Jewish, would never eat non-kosher meat. But she'd been alone in the house. It had to have been her. One night before Passover, she gorged on jars of pickles and olives, consuming so much vinegar white spots sprouted up along her hands. Another time she ate a dozen raw eggs and became dreadfully ill. After her nightly binges, she'd throw up in her sleep, leaving her husband to change the soiled sheets. Sometimes John found her sitting up in bed with food still in her mouth. He child-proofed the fridge, so Makinen set her sights on the pantry, eating cans of soft, cold vegetables. Makinen refitted her bedroom doorknob so that the lock was on the outside of the door. When she was unable to turn the handle, Makinen sleepwalked her way onto the porch and into the kitchen. "Nothing was going to stop me from eating," she said.

Consuming thousands of calories a night, Makinen's five foot, one-hundred-pound frame gained sixty pounds. She stopped eating during the day, petrified by her nocturnal hunger. Then in 2004, after six years of eating her way through the night, she Googled "sleep" and "eating" and found a message board of Ambien users whose stories were eerily familiar. People were gorging themselves on anything their sleeping hands could shove into their mouths.

Makinen contacted Susan Chana Lask, a high-profile New York attorney who received thousands of calls, letters, and emails from Ambien users who were suffering like Makinen, sleepwalking their way into all different kinds of trouble. When we spoke, Lask shared some people's experiences while taking the drug. After three nights taking Ambien, a financial analyst from Texas awoke on the cold concrete floor of a jail cell. She had crashed her mother's vehicle into two parked cars and left the scene to return to her bedroom, where she was later arrested. A lieutenant in the U.S. Navy based in Tampa, Florida, was arrested for shoplifting on and off the base and had no recollection of the thefts.

In 2006, Lask filed a class action lawsuit against Sanofi-Aventis to warn consumers of Ambien's possible side effects. "When consumers contacted me about Ambien putting them into a dreamlike hypnotic state where they wildly drove cars and committed crimes with no memory of their actions," Lask told me, "I made it my mission to fight for proper warnings on that drug by commencing a class action."

Lask considered the class action a victory and closed it in one year. Her highly publicized case had brought attention to the risks of the sleep drug, and the consumer warnings that she advocated for were implemented for Ambien and similar sleep medications.[7] On March 14, 2007, the U.S. Food and Drug Administration urged companies that make sedative-hypnotic sleep medications to "strengthen their product labeling to include stronger language concerning potential risks. These risks include . . . complex sleep-related behaviors, which may include sleep driving."[8]

The many years of sleep eating had taken its toll on Makinen's health. She had developed an ulcer, GERD, and acid reflux disease. With the help of her doctor, Makinen weaned herself off Ambien and onto Lunesta, another sleep aid, and stopped walking and eating in her sleep.

Around this time, my research led me to the work of the late Mark Mahowald, who extensively studied parasomnias and, over his long career in sleep medicine and research, made significant contributions to their diagnosis and treatment. When I spoke with Mahowald, I asked about Ambien's possible side effect of sleep eating. "Everyone points to Ambien, but Ambien is probably an artifact of prescribing practices," he explained. When we spoke in 2006, he pointed out there were more than 26 million prescriptions for Ambien in the United States that year, which made it one of the most widely prescribed sedatives. "Therefore, that's probably why it's the one most frequently associated with sleepwalking, sleep eating, and sleep driving," he explained.

We talked about how the sleep aid Halcion was banned in Britain in the early nineties with many reports of amnesia among users. In some reports, people would board a transatlantic flight, take the sleeping pill, then get off the plane and wander around, later having little or no memory of what they had done. How was this possible?

Mahowald pointed to the fact that sleep is not a whole brain phenomenon. There is different brain activity at different sleep stages. All parasomnias are intrusion of one brain state into another, he said. During sleepwalking, part of the brain is awake enough to perform complex tasks like eating. At the same time, parts of the brain involved in monitoring and awareness have quieted down. In the field of sleep, this is known as state dissociation, said Mahowald. It's like a switch that gets stuck, he explained.

Generally speaking, a sedative hypnotic can predispose someone to a mixture of brain states. Many sleep medications cause amnesia and sleep, and sleep is an amnesic state, he said. So the likelihood of sleepwalking while taking a sleeping pill is greater than the chance of this occurring spontaneously.

It was interesting to consider that there aren't more reports of parasomnia behaviour. "When you think of the millions of people sleeping every night, switching from wake to REM to non-REM, on and off throughout the night, these things don't happen very often," said Mahowald. "You would think these switching errors would happen much more frequently than they do."

The One Thing That Nobody Can Fake

THERE HAVE BEEN REPORTS of "indecent exposure" during sleep since the early nineteenth century, and researchers have been writing about the connection between parasomnias and sexual activity for decades. In 2007, sexsomnia was recognized as a medical condition by the International Classification of Sleep Disorders. Yet it often goes undiagnosed.

One study found that 96 percent of participants with sexsomnia had total amnesia for their sexual encounter during sleep.[9] Like Luedecke, most people don't try to cover up their actions and often become upset when they discover what they have done.[10] What complicates matters is a sharp spike in sexsomnia defences for sexual assault. I spoke with independent sleep expert Neil Stanley, who has provided testimony on many sexsomnia cases. He has noticed an increase in reported cases and now hears at least one case a month. When I asked him what might have led to the increase, Stanley pointed to the fact that sexsomnia is a condition that many people don't understand, including some judges and juries. I didn't have a firm grasp on the sleep disorder, either.

It is a huge concern that defendants will falsely claim the condition, Stanley said. "I strongly suspect there are people out there who are as guilty as anything," he told me. "But they're just trying this defence." Stanley pointed out that even if someone has sleep-related behaviours characteristic of this parasomnia when they're run in a lab, this isn't proof that the same behaviours happened during an incident in question. I was struck by the costly consequences of a sleep disorder many people had never even heard of. This dominoed into one question after another. How could the courts be sure that someone had the condition? Could they be certain that someone had a parasomnia attack outside of a sleep lab? Could it be faked? How was this avoidable?

I needed to learn more about the condition and how it was evaluated and diagnosed. So I met with sleep expert and physician Colin Shapiro, who coined the term sexsomnia in 2003 after he observed a number of patients with sexual behaviour in their sleep. I spent a Sunday morning with Shapiro at his Toronto home, trying to unravel some of the mysteries around parasominas.

"If you talk in your sleep, nobody cares. If you sing in your sleep, it's not so serious. But if you interfere with somebody, then it is." If this happens in a relationship, a partner may find the behaviour odd and out of character, added Shapiro. I asked Shapiro about the Luedecke case. At the trial, Shapiro had been called as the expert witness by the defence. Was Luedecke suffering from sexsomnia?

At the time of the trial, Shapiro examined some contributing factors: Luedecke's brother experienced mini-awakenings during deep sleep; Luedecke used to sleepwalk as a child and there were other instances in which he'd woken to find himself having sex with a girlfriend. Shapiro identified possible triggers for the attack in question. Luedecke had been severely sleep-deprived, having been awake for twenty-two hours; he'd consumed more than sixteen alcoholic drinks at the croquet party; he was exhausted from his physically demanding job as a landscaper; and he had mourned several recent deaths. Stress, sleep deprivation, alcohol, and physical exhaustion would have wreaked havoc on his sleep cycle and increased his amount of deep sleep, giving him ample opportunity to have a parasomnia attack.

Luedecke spent two nights in the sleep lab to determine whether he had what Shapiro calls the "hallmark of parasomnia": an abrupt arousal during deep sleep. In the lab, Luedecke's brain waves, respiration, and heart rate were recorded, and he was videotaped while he slept. While Luedecke fell asleep, a technician watched him move through light and intermediate sleep. Once he dipped into a period of deep sleep, he had a sudden brief arousal. In fact, there were several hiccups of brain activity scrawled across his sleep record during the night, and at one point, Luedecke's eyes flicked open, and he began to mumble something incoherent and wave his arm about strangely. Then within ninety seconds, he was asleep again.

There it was, scrawled across his sleep record: the sudden, unexpected arousal from deep sleep. Shapiro sees it as a thumbprint or signature of a parasomnia. It's the one thing that nobody can fake, Shapiro explained during the Luedecke trial. A person can't will themselves to have this feature. They can't suppress it, either.[11] If this happens in a sleep lab, it shows that someone has the capacity to have these sudden arousals from deep sleep, explained Shapiro.

Shapiro examined the details of the specific night in question. He knew that Luedecke had fallen asleep around 4 a.m. and L.O. had found him on top of her about thirty to sixty minutes later, a time that he was likely to be in deep sleep. Shapiro noted that the incident took place in the living room in front of several witnesses, an unusual place to commit a sexual assault. Luedecke didn't try to conceal his identity. There was no history of sexual misconduct. In L.O.'s statement to the police, she described Luedecke as someone who had just woken from a sound sleep. After the incident, Luedecke surrendered voluntarily to the police, which in the physician's experience is "very typical" of sexsomniacs.[12] He didn't seem to be concealing anything. Shapiro was convinced that Luedecke suffered from sexsomnia.

Justice R.J. Otter concluded that Luedecke was in an "automatistic state" characteristic of sexsomnia. Yet a contentious question remained: whether Luedecke's condition was a mental disorder, which is defined by the Criminal Code as a "disease of the mind."[13] The judge had to determine whether a normal person would have had the same "automatistic reaction" as Luedecke. Shapiro explained to the court that a parasomnia does not really have a pathology. It is a condition that arises from the normal process of sleep. Every one of us descends from light sleep into a period of deep sleep throughout the night, and it is during this normal process that something goes wrong.

Considering sexsomnia a mental illness is "very bad news," said Shapiro. This type of parasomnia has the same brain activity as sleepwalking, another type of NREM parasomnia. "If they call sexsomnia a disease of the mind," said Shapiro, "every four-year-old who gets up and walks in his sleep has got a disease of the mind, and that would be a pretty dangerous path to go down." A landmark Supreme Court of Canada case, *R v. Parks*, considered whether sleepwalking could be classified as a disease of the mind.

"It's All My Fault."

IN THE SPRING OF 1987, Ken Parks found himself in a mess of trouble. The twenty-three-year-old had a gambling problem; he had emptied his savings and to fund his bets on horse races, and he had embezzled more than $30,000 from his employer. Parks lost his job and faced criminal charges. He couldn't find work and his wife became the sole provider for the young couple and their infant daughter. His wife was supportive during this difficult time. Parks was close to his in-laws, Barbara Ann and Denis Woods. Barbara Ann called him the "gentle giant." They knew of his financial trouble and had invited him to dinner to talk about it.

The night before, his wife returned from work a few minutes before 11 p.m. They chatted for a while before she went to bed. Parks stayed on the couch in the living room, where he watched TV and eventually fell asleep. In the early morning, Parks got into his car and drove more than twenty kilometres to his in-laws. If he took his usual route, he would have navigated on and off the highway, through eight sets of traffic lights and around six turns. Parks had a key to his in-laws' house, which he visited often. This particular night, he parked in an underground lot, removed a tire iron from his car, and let himself into the dark house.

Once inside, he went to the kitchen to retrieve a knife before making his way to his in-laws' bedroom. The couple was fast asleep. Parks went over to Denis and straddled the man. He wrapped his large hands around his father-in-law's neck and strangled him until he was unconscious. Parks then turned to Barbara, whom he beat with a blunt object, likely the tire iron that was later found in the bedroom. He fractured the woman's skull and she suffered a brain hemorrhage. Parks stabbed his mother-in-law several times, penetrating her heart, diaphragm, stomach, and lung. Armed with the kitchen knife, Parks left the house and drove to a local police station. His hands were severely cut when he entered the station and said, "I just killed someone with my bare hands. . . . My God, I've just killed two people. My hands . . . I've just killed my mother- and father-in-law. I stabbed and beat them to death. It's all my fault."[14] While Barbara died, Denis was hospitalized and recovered.

His memories of the incident were hazy and confusing. He could picture his mother-in-law's face, which he described as a "help me face, a sad face."[15] Parks recalled thinking that he needed to get help. He had an image of a knife in his hand, and he thought that Barbara might be dead because she was silent in his memory. He couldn't recall seeing his father-in-law. Parks thought that it must all have been a dream. Roger Broughton, a sleep expert who testified in the Parks case, explained that it is completely possible to do something while sleepwalking and have no understanding of the consequences of your actions. When asked if Parks would have been able to stop what he was doing, Broughton told the court, "I think it would all have been an unconscious activity, uncontrolled and unmediated."

Parks was charged with first-degree murder and attempted murder. As in the Luedecke case, there was no dispute over who committed the crime. What was being determined was the state of mind that the defendant was in when he attacked his in-laws. At the time of the incident, Parks was sleep-deprived and stressed out. He came from a family of poor sleepers who had nightmares and walked and talked in their sleep. He got on well with his in-laws, who wanted to help him through his recent financial troubles.

Parks' defence was that he was in a state of non-insane automatism brought on by sleepwalking when he committed the crime. It had to be decided whether sleepwalking should be considered a "disease of the mind." The expert witnesses called by the defence were in agreement that Parks was sleepwalking when the horrible incident occurred. They went on to explain that the sleep problem is not a neurological or psychiatric illness. And they concluded that Parks was not suffering from a mental disorder. The court learned that a sleepwalker does not have the ability to think or act voluntarily and cannot carry out a plan that was devised when they were awake.

Parks was acquitted of first degree and attempted murder. The case went to the Court of Appeal, which upheld the acquittal. When the case went to the Supreme Court of Canada, Parks's acquittal was again upheld. Sleep-walking was considered non-insane automatism, and Parks was found not guilty.

In the Luedecke case, Judge Otter deliberated over a possible disease of the mind and Luedecke's danger to society. The judge returned to the court with his verdict. He pointed out this was a rare case. The judge was satisfied that at the time of the event, the defendant was "in a state of non-insane automatism. His conduct was not voluntary."[16] Luedecke was acquitted of sexual assault. The Crown appealed the decision. In 2008, the Ontario Court of Appeal upheld the acquittal. Luedecke was free of the charges.

I discovered that when people act out their dreams, they are in a mysterious mixed brain state that bridges waking and sleep. They get stuck in between the waking and dreaming worlds as parts of their brain quiet down while other parts buzz with activity. When their rational, conscious mind comes back online, it begins the natural process of piecing together a story from a jumble of thoughts and images. The question swirls around their mind: What is reality, and what is a dream?

I shifted my focus back to everyday dreams to explore how our dream stories reflect our current state of mind. As our psychological well-being changes, so do our dreams. Possibly the best example happens to be one of the most interesting times in dream research. A time when we discovered the intrinsic connection between our mental health and the world around us and, inevitably, our dreams.

The COVID-19 global pandemic offered researchers a natural experiment in dreaming as people's anxieties and fixations with an unknown and invisible threat moved through the waking and dreaming worlds. We were isolated, disconnected, and at many times afraid, and our dreams told the story.

Chapter Four

Dreams and Our
Mental Health

IN MARCH 2020, THE WORLD HEALTH ORGANIZATION DECLARED the COVID-19 global pandemic. Overnight, the world adopted a new vocabulary and way of life. In everyday conversation, we talked about sheltering in place and lockdowns, N95 masks and six feet of separation. We were told to stay home. Only leave when it was absolutely necessary. We moved cautiously among masked faces, trying to smile with the crinkle of our eyes. We were alone together. Confined by the increasing claustrophobia of our homes, of the same monotonous routine. "Going out" consisted of a trip to the grocery store. It was a strange dichotomy of boredom and fear. We lived *Groundhog Day* under the constant threat of an invisible, deadly virus.

As the world around us contracted, our dream world broke wide open. Dreams became more vivid, bizarre, and emotionally charged.[1] Untethered from new daily constraints, our dreaming minds were free to explore the pandemic in abstract and unusual ways. We tested out strange scenarios, practiced skills like mask fitting and social distancing, and tried to escape from new threats brought on by the pandemic.[2]

The pandemic proved to be an ideal entryway into my research on dreams and mental health. There were countless studies on pandemic dreams, and as I read accounts from dreamers around the world, I began to remember my own bizarre dreams at a time when the waking world had shut its doors only to burst open the alternate realm of dreams. It was easy to get caught up in other people's dreams. I was fascinated to see how they explored the same themes that ran through my own nightly stories. But first, I wanted to understand why COVID-19 had such an effect on our dream life. Was it simply because our dreams reflected what we were thinking about and doing during the day? As I sifted through databases of pandemic dream studies, I focused on three main reasons why COVID-19 made such an impression on our dreams.

First, I looked at the pandemic's sudden impact on our sleeping habits. Working from home, we switched off our alarms, went to bed later, and woke up naturally. More sleep time equaled more dream time, which often included an extra period of early morning REM sleep, when we have some of our most vivid dreams. If we woke up during REM and lingered in bed, there was a chance we would remember these intense dreams that seemed to be telling us so much. Yet extra time in bed didn't mean a better night's rest. For many of us, sleep quality deteriorated during the pandemic. We tossed and turned our way to sleep and woke up throughout the night.

Sleep is inherently tied to mental health, which offered a second reason why the pandemic changed our dreams. When we are stressed, anxious, or depressed, our sleep as well as our dreams suffer, increasing our chances of having bad dreams and nightmares. During the COVID-19 pandemic, we faced the greatest threat to mental health since the Second World War, explained Adrian James, the president of the United Kingdom's Royal College of Psychiatrists.[3] We battled a collective crisis as well as our own personal struggles. Our fight-or-flight response was on high alert, fraying our mental fabric. This made us deeply aware of how our environment affects our mental health, which influences our dreams. Some of us developed new mental health issues while others struggled with existing challenges.[4]

One study early in the pandemic examined the connection between sleep quality and mental health during the "I stay home" order issued by the Italian government in March 2020. The researchers tested whether people's stress, anxiety, and depression levels affected their sleep quality and sleep habits. It was a large study, with more than 6,500 adults completing an online survey that assessed their sleep and mental health. More than half of the Italian subjects had poor sleep quality and sleep habits, and this was related to increased psychological distress during quarantine.[5]

The researchers discovered that certain people were more at risk for poor sleep, including women, those who had lost a loved one to the COVID-19 virus, and participants who were struggling with severe stress, anxiety, and depression. This validated the findings of other studies that showed the bidirectional relationship between sleep and stress.[6] I thought about how stress wreaks havoc on my sleep. And if I don't sleep, my stress level soars. Sleepless nights tend to leave an unsettling feeling the next day when it seems hard to cope with even the smallest problems.

Our frequent awakenings offered a silver lining for dream research: more opportunity for people to remember and share their dreams. Dream recall spiked early in the pandemic. One study found that 29 percent of participants remembered more of their dreams in early May of 2020.[7] As dream researcher Tore Nielsen explained, "As a dream 'event,' the pandemic is unprecedented."[8] Researchers could study the sleep effects of a global crisis when people were confined to their homes, sleeping longer and more fitfully, and spending more time online. It was a chance to study dreams during a global emergency in the era of virtual connection and physical separation. Dream reports flooded chat groups and social media as people tried to make sense of their dreams. It didn't take long for #pandemicdreams and #covidnightmares to go viral.

Idreamofcovid.com was launched early in the pandemic by Erin Gravley. Ten days into the San Francisco Bay Area's shelter-in-place order, Gravley dreamt of people social distancing. Her dream characters avoided shaking hands and stayed away from one another. It was remarkable how quickly her dreams reflected her new reality. She had read *The Third Reich of Dreams* by Charlotte Beradt and was curious to see how dreams would express our shared anxieties and experiences. Idreamofcovid.com was a place for people to share their dreams. Erin's sister, Grace, created sketches to accompany dream reports, offering visuals for strange and often terrifying dreams.

One of the earliest patterns that Erin noticed was dreamers associating hugging with danger. Dreamers became frightened as someone tried to hug them, yelling things like "You're hurting me; you're going to kill me."[9] Another recurrent theme was windows. Grace wondered if it was related to a feeling of being trapped. Dreamers would peer out at something frightening or watch the virus seep in through a window. Then there was a collective obsession with hygiene. Dreamers attempted to scrub surfaces clean or became upset by people eating with their hands.

Our sudden and strange new way of life offered a third possible reason why the pandemic changed our dreams. Research shows that dreams express our waking experiences, thoughts, and emotions. During the pandemic, we focused on washing our hands, scrubbing surfaces, and ensuring our masks fit properly. Not only did we dream about forgetting or losing our masks, we dreamt about our thoughts and feelings around this suddenly ubiquitous object in our pockets and attached to our wrists, leaving its mark on the faces of front-line workers.

What tipped the odds of dreaming about the pandemic even further was its impact on our lives. In a May 2020 study, more than three thousand Americans responded to an online dream survey. Dream researchers Kelly Bulkeley and Michael Schredl tested whether the impact of COVID-19 on people's lives resulted in negative or pandemic-related dreams. If your mental or physical health or social life was greatly affected by the pandemic, did this make you have bad dreams or COVID-related dreams? At the time of the study, the United States had more than 1 million confirmed cases of COVID-19 and around eighty thousand COVID-related deaths.[10] It was a time of online school, restricted travel, and cancelled events.

The more people were affected by the pandemic, namely their mental health, the more their dreams were affected. This included more dream recall, COVID-related dreams, and negative dreams. The study found that women and young people with higher education were more affected by COVID-19. Interestingly, the majority of subjects who reported health-related dreams had health-related worries but didn't necessarily have health problems.

The findings supported the idea that we can use our dreams to assess our mental health. If we are having more negative dreams, this could indicate that our mental health is at risk or suffering, especially during times of crisis. Dreams indicate how we are feeling. At the same time, they tell us how our "natural healing resources" are responding to what's happening, explained Bulkeley when we spoke. In this way, dreams act as an emotional gauge that indicates how we are coping at the moment. Recurrent bad dreams or nightmares are our internal warning system raising a red flag, telling us to attend to our mental health.

I spoke with Schredl to better understand what dreams can reveal about our mental health. He explained that it is important to look at a series of dreams rather than a single dream to determine how we are coping. "It could be a very different assessment if you look at only one dream," said Schredl, head of research at the Central Institute of Mental Health sleep laboratory in Mannheim, Germany. He pointed out there can be great variability from dream to dream. In a single night, you can have a calm and comforting dream followed by a terrifying nightmare. Viewed in isolation, each of these dreams would create a very different picture of a person's state of mind. Even if someone is stress-free and healthy, they can still have the occasional nightmare. Then there is the complicating factor of which dreams we remember. What if we only recall bad dreams? It's beneficial to look at a series of dreams to identify patterns and connect the frequency of negative dreams with what is happening in waking life. "There is a direct correlation between the emotional state in your waking life and the average emotional state in your dream life," explained Schredl.

During times of crisis, dreams often reveal our collective anxieties and coping mechanisms. The COVID-19 pandemic changed what we dreamt about as well as the quantity and quality of our dream sleep. I discovered that the pandemic's effect on our dream content had similarities and stark contrasts to other times of crisis. I spoke with dream researcher and psychologist Deirdre Barrett, who has been studying the effects of personal and global crises on dreams for decades. "Any really strong, immediate threat tends to get our attention prioritized over strong, positive things," explained Barrett.

The assistant professor of psychology at Harvard Medical School has studied dreams after 9/11, dreams of Kuwaitis during the first Gulf War, and POWs living in concentration camps during the Second World War. She told me how 9/11 was a kind of "one-time event" that was very immediate and threatening. Many people directly affected by the terrorist attacks, including first responders, people who escaped from the Twin Towers, and those in the streets who witnessed people fall from the burning buildings, suffered from post-traumatic nightmares with dream content that stayed very close to actual experiences. A classic PTSD nightmare "can have some surreal elements and be a little dreamlike," said Barrett. "But it will usually just be a replay with some variation."

Another group that suffered from nightmares after 9/11 were those with past trauma. Barrett identified "hybrid dreams" that combined elements related to 9/11 with a person's traumatic history. Barrett gave the example of a woman who dreamt that she was on a plane and recognized the man who sexually assaulted her when she was a teenager. The man had a box cutter and was going to crash the plane. Barrett found the data set for 9/11 had more in common with data sets from brief, dramatic natural disasters like hurricanes and tornadoes that played out an immediacy related to people's fears. Pandemic dreams imagined an entirely different kind of fear.

In the early days of the COVID-19 pandemic, the virus often showed up in dreams as this invisible entity creeping toward people. The long-term, encroaching threat of COVID resulted in images that Barrett had not seen in other crises or trauma data sets. There weren't necessarily terrifying images like attackers with box cutters or buildings crumbling to the ground. Instead, it was more of what the unconscious came up with to visualize something that was, by its very nature, invisible, said Barrett.

People dreamt of invisible monsters and sketched many variations on this unseen, looming threat. One person dreamt of walking in a dimly lit space where all they could see was the monster's shadow. Another dreamer heard a monster's footsteps behind them while someone else watched people falling as bites were taken out of them. Then an invisible creature attacked someone else within six feet, offering a strange incorporation of the social distancing rule during the pandemic. Suddenly, the person realized that they were within six feet of someone else who had just died. As they felt the monster land on them, they awoke.

Another common topic was bugs, which Barrett connected with the slang term for virus or infection. While there were a couple of giant insects in her data set, the majority featured dreams of swarming insects. There were cockroaches racing toward someone or "masses of toxic wiggly worms," said Barrett. The data sets for 9/11 and the POWs during the Second World War didn't include insect dreams, which she believed were unique to COVID being an infection.

As the pandemic progressed and people were exposed to disturbing images of patients in the ICU and makeshift mortuaries to manage the overwhelming number of deaths, COVID-related dream images became more concrete. Many people struggled with the fear of catching the virus or were in a constant state of panic as they wondered if they in fact had COVID-19, and they put their own dreamy twist on the common theme. In her book *Pandemic Dreams*, Barrett shared how one dreamer's COVID screening test came in the form of a pregnancy test while another person had to take a multiple-choice exam to see if they had the virus. Fear manifested in various scenarios, from being unable to find a hospital to noticing that a syringe was labeled "cyanide" just as someone was about to receive an injection. Such dreams highlighted our sense of vulnerability during the pandemic, explained Barrett.[11]

For her book on COVID dreams, Barrett collected over 9,000 dreams from more than 3,700 people around the world. She used an online survey to connect with dreamers during the COVID-19 pandemic and compiled their dream reports, and she discovered some fascinating findings compared to dreams during other crises.

In five hundred dream reports from POWs in the Second World War, Barrett found that soldiers dreamt of being home again, seeing friends and eating their favourite foods. During the pandemic, some reported dreams involved birthday parties with lots of people or sheltering in place with a former romantic partner.[12]

During other crises, Barrett found that certain threats in people's waking lives were carried out in their dreams. She described a Kuwaiti woman who witnessed Iraqi soldiers press a gun to her children's heads. In the mother's dream, the soldiers fired the gun.[13] After the attack on the Twin Towers, a man who worked in the World Trade Center and was reunited with his wife dreamt that he found her among the dead.

Barrett discovered that many health care workers during the COVID-19 pandemic dreamt of being unable to save their patients. In one dream, a ventilator transformed into a water cooler as a doctor tried to help a patient. An Italian anesthesiologist dreamt he administered medication to sedate a patient, lost his balance, and fell out the window, taking his patient with him. The anesthesiologist survived the fall, upset and ashamed that his patient had died.[14] Just as first responders and rescue crews battled nightmares after the traumatic events of 9/11, front-line workers during the pandemic struggled with post-traumatic nightmares, reliving an endless battle to try and protect patients from the deadly virus.

As the pandemic progressed, there were more concrete dreams that reflected our daily routines. Unlike other crises, the COVID pandemic had an effect on all of us. We weren't only witnessing the distressing event on television. We were also living it. By late March and April of 2020, many of us dreamt of staying six feet apart, wearing a mask, and obsessively washing our hands. This made me wonder if these dreams were related to the idea that dreams help us practice new skills and consolidate memories.

Dream researchers discovered that the pandemic affected some people's dreams more than others. Women and young people suffered from more nightmares during the pandemic.[15] Women made up the majority of health care and front-line workers, unpaid caregivers and victims of gender-based violence. Young people suffered as they lost important milestones to the pandemic as schools and activities closed for months on end.

People with more stress, anxiety, and depression during lockdown had more bad dreams, COVID-related dreams, and nightmares.[16] It was a domino effect as our environment affected our mental health, which shaped our dreams. Add the impact of a shared traumatic event to our own personal stresses, and you have what pandemic dreams were made of.

Now that I understood how COVID-19 turned our dream lives upside down, I widened my lens to everyday dreams to examine their connection to mental health. I looked at dreams of the general population as well as dreams of individuals with mental health conditions like anxiety, depression, and PTSD. As I made my way through a tower of scientific studies, I focused on three aspects of the relationship between dreams and mental health: what dreams reveal about our mental health; how our dreams change with our psychological well-being; and why it's often impossible to hide from our worries and preoccupations, even in our dreams.

For decades, Antonio Zadra has studied many dimensions of dreaming, including the relationship between dreams and our psychological well-being. It all began with an intense and hyperreal dream in college that changed the course of his life.

Here We Go Again

ONE NIGHT WHEN HE was in college in Montreal, Zadra dreamt he was convicted of a crime and sent to prison, where he was stabbed by another inmate.[17] Then Zadra ran across the prison yard and scaled a barbed wire fence without a scratch. Safe on the other side, he noticed something peculiar. He stood in a field of snow, yet the prison yard was covered in grass. Miraculously, his stab wounds had healed. Zadra realized that it must all be a dream. He scooped up some snow, packing it into a snowball, and was amazed by the cold sensation in his hands. He yelled at someone and marveled at how loud his voice was in his dream while his body was asleep in bed. He threw a snowball at a man who threatened to punch him. Zadra panicked, forgetting that it was a dream. Then he met another man, who tried to convince Zadra that what he was experiencing wasn't a dream. It was mind-boggling how vivid and real everything looked. Zadra awoke to the fascinating world of dreams.

Today, Zadra is a professor of psychology at the Université de Montréal and a dream researcher at the Centre for Advanced Research in Sleep Medicine in Montreal. Zadra studies many facets of dreams, including recurrent dreams and nightmares. Recurrent dreams can tell us a lot about our well-being. These repetitive dreams revisit a "remembered experience."[18] It might be the theme that is repeated or, in some cases, the dream plot. Some recurrent dreams stay relatively close to the same story while other dreams offer wild variations. Some of us have had the same recurrent dream since we were kids.

I was about five years old when I first dreamt that I was balancing along the top beam of a metal scaffolding. Every time I have this recurrent dream, I picture it like the rusted bones of an abandoned warehouse. I walk along the thin metal scaffolding like a gymnast on a balance beam, guiding one foot in front of the other while staring into the dark night. I try to focus on what's in front of me. Then something compels me to look down. My dream world begins to spin. At some point, I stumble and begin falling through the darkness. Just as I'm about to hit the ground, I bolt awake. I've had this dream on and off all my life. It's the same basic plot. At some point in my teens, my dream-self transformed from a five-year-old girl to my actual age. Every few years, I imagine I'm that little girl again, but mostly I picture myself as an adult, falling helplessly into the unknown.

Falling is a common theme in recurrent dreams. So is being chased, attempting to drive a car that is out of control, and taking an exam, although we put our own spin on the details. Zadra shared his recurrent exam dreams that explore the same theme through different variations. One variation has a government official tell Zadra that their records indicate he didn't show up for an exam, which is usually in physics or math. He must retake the exam the next morning. If he doesn't pass, all of his studies to this point will be voided. Some people might dream of being late or unprepared for an exam, while others might sit down to take the exam only to find that its pages are blank.

In a 2006 study, Zadra and other dream researchers found that approximately 85 percent of recurrent dreams were negative. In about 40 percent of the recurrent dreams, the dreamer was in danger. This included being chased, frantically searching for a place to hide, or watching helplessly as they were threatened with injury or death.[19]

A recent study found that people living with anxiety disorders tended to have different dreams than healthy subjects. Anton Rimish and Reinhard Pietrowsky discovered that people experiencing anxiety had more characters, social and aggressive interactions, and negative emotions in their dreams. The subjects dreamt of more failures, misfortunes, and threatening situations. Subjects with an anxiety disorder had several common themes running through their dreams, including being chased, physically attacked, frozen with fright, and feeling anxious about other people's aggressive actions.[20] While studies indicate that only about 10 percent of recurrent dreams are positive, they can be the source of wonder for dreamers.

Carl Jung had a powerful dream that helped him conceive of the collective unconscious that lay beneath the personal unconscious, connecting each of us with humanity. In 1909, Jung was on a steamship headed for the United States with Sigmund Freud, who at the time was his mentor and friend. During the voyage, Jung dreamt that he was in an unfamiliar house that he somehow felt was his own.

Jung's famous house dream began with him in the salon that was located on the second floor of the house. This could be seen as his personal unconscious. Then Jung descended to the ground floor, where it was quite dark and everything around him was from the fifteenth or sixteenth century. Jung explored the house and found a heavy door that led to a stone stairway. He descended into the cellar and found himself in an ancient, vaulted room. He opened one of the stone slabs on the floor, revealing another stairway. He followed the narrow stone steps into a cave with bones and bits of pottery strewn across the floor. He imagined the lower levels symbolizing the collective unconscious. Jung's dream house gave him a structure for the human psyche.[21] In this way, exploring a house in our dreams is like exploring our mind, including our thoughts, emotions, and motivations. One idea is that discovering a new room can symbolize uncovering a new part of ourselves.

Recurrent dreams don't seem to happen randomly. In the late 1970s, pioneering dream researcher Rosalind Cartwright, known as the Queen of Dreams by her peers, conducted several studies on recurrent dreams. She found that repetitive dreams occurred during times of stress. If the recurrent dream stopped, it might indicate that the person had resolved the conflict in their mind and was better able to cope with their waking situation.[22]

About a decade later, Ronald J. Brown and D. C. Donderi performed a well-documented study on the connection between recurrent dreams and psychological well-being. Their goal was to test whether a recurrent dream signified an unresolved conflict, and if the unfinished issue was associated with a lower level of well-being. They found that people with recurrent dreams had more anxious and conflict-oriented dreams, and this experience affected their psychological well-being. Yet none of the subjects sought help from a mental health professional. The group of past recurrent dreamers, those who no longer had recurrent dreams, had significantly higher levels of well-being compared to recurrent dreamers. The benefit of overcoming recurrent dreams didn't end there. The study found that past recurrent dreamers had statistically higher well-being than people who didn't experience recurrent dreams. This reflected Jung's assertion that if we resolved a psychological conflict, our recurrent dreams about this conflict would end, improving our psychological well-being.[23]

In a 2006 study, Zadra and Nicholas Pesant examined the relationship between everyday dreams and psychological well-being at fixed points in time as well as over the course of many years. The study highlighted the importance of studying a series of dreams. Often, we think about a dream in isolation. We might ask ourselves what a dream could mean or wonder why we're dreaming it at a certain point in our lives. Is it trying to tell us something? While it can be informative to look at a specific dream, this is only part of the dream story. Examining a series of dreams over time lets us identify patterns and parallels between our waking and dreaming lives. Maybe someone is going through a divorce or struggling with the loss of a loved one. Their dreams over time might reveal how they are dealing with these ongoing personal stressors. Examining only a single dream would be the same as looking at an event in isolation.

Zadra and I discussed how it would be quite unusual for someone to go to a therapist and talk only about what had happened within say an hour of a particular day. Maybe a person was hit with a panic attack while they were on the subway. To better understand the situation, they might want to look for context. What was happening leading up to the panic attack? Was it a one-time occurrence or had it happened before? We can do the same with our dreams. Looking at dreams over time gives us a broader perspective on their possible significance. We can see if a certain dream theme has popped up before. Or maybe we have a recurrent dream when we are stressed.

Take Zadra's exam dreams as an example. Zadra noticed his recurrent dreams popped up at certain times. "They tended to come when I had some self-doubts about anything," he said. "It could be academic work, family life, whatever, but in periods of self-doubt. And that's a great metaphor." An exam is designed to test our competency. In dreams, we work through this theme in creative ways, exploring our feelings of self-doubt. It can be enlightening to examine which dream themes we explore at certain times.

The Power of Positive Thoughts

I LEARNED THAT DREAMS reveal when our mental health is declining in day-to-day life as well as during times of crisis. It made me wonder, what about the reverse? What can dreams reveal about our well-being? I took another look at Zadra and Pesant's study on dreams and psychological well-being. They recruited men and women between the ages of thirty and ninety and analyzed their dreams at certain points as well as over time. They looked at the frequency of positive and negative dreams, friendly and aggressive interactions, and instances of success and good fortune and failure and misfortune. Then they measured psychological well-being at different times.

At fixed points as well as across time, there was a relationship between people's self-reported well-being and the emotions and content of their dreams. People who reported lower well-being had more negative emotions and aggressive interactions in their dreams. Remarkably, when people's psychological well-being changed, the emotions and content of their dreams changed accordingly. So when their well-being deteriorated, their dreams became more negative. When people's well-being improved, they had more positive dreams. This showed how connected dreams are to our psychological well-being.[24]

In a way, this connection makes us empowered dreamers. If we can achieve a state of well-being, this can lead to positive dreams. A positive outlook during the day might lead to a positive dream life. Of course, finding and maintaining well-being isn't easy. It's difficult to understand let alone boost well-being. The more I read about well-being, the more I got tangled up in its complexities. Well-being doesn't just cover the absence of mental health challenges. We aren't necessarily satisfied with our lives or feel a sense of peace and harmony simply because we're not experiencing anxiety or depression at a particular moment. There are different types and components of well-being that affect our waking and dreaming states of mind.

Hedonic well-being involves how positively or negatively we think about our lives. This includes how we perceive our work, personal relationships, and health. It's a subjective form of well-being that reflects how satisfied we are with life. Eudaimonic well-being focuses on meaning and purpose in life. It's about personal growth and reaching our potential as a human being. While these concepts were mostly developed by Western culture, there is another central aspect to well-being that is rooted in many Eastern philosophies, including Buddhism, Hinduism, and Taoism.[25] Inner peace and harmony are integral to well-being. Peace of mind elicits feelings of satisfaction and contentment. It's not about experiencing constant excitement or positivity. This facet of well-being centres around finding acceptance and peace even when there are difficulties in life. This is where dreams come in.

In a recent study, psychology and neuroscience researcher Pilleriin Sikka and a group of researchers investigated the relationship between dreams and different aspects of well-being. Specifically, they wanted to test whether people's dreams were influenced by peace of mind. Healthy subjects completed a well-being questionnaire and kept a dream journal for three weeks, rating their dream emotions. The dream researchers found that peace of mind was related to positive dreams. Conversely, anxiety was associated with negative dreams. A positive as well as a negative state of mind had the power to shape people's dreams. This supported the idea that dream reports can be used as markers of mental health, indicating well-being as well as ill-being.

It can be hard to fall asleep when thoughts or concerns are weighing on your mind. What if you could stop those negative thoughts? Would this affect your sleep? These questions led me to a recent study on the relationship between rumination and sleep. I spoke with Andrew Gall, who, along with colleagues, investigated whether negative rumination makes sleep worse, and if a negative effect could be reversed with compassionate reappraisal. They gathered 180 undergraduate students for the two-night study. Before bed on the first night, subjects thought about a time when they were hurt or offended by someone. The issue had to be unresolved, and they focused on their negative thoughts and feelings about the event. Then they spent some time writing about how the person hurt them.

"The individuals are upset. They are angry," said Gall, an associate professor of psychology at Hope College in Michigan. "They're in a state that they're not very forgiving toward the person." That night, their sleep quality was measured, including how long it took to fall asleep and how many times they awoke during the night. There was a significant effect on people's sleep. They tossed and turned, taking longer to fall asleep. They had trouble staying asleep and woke up more during the night. In the morning, they had more intrusive thoughts about the upsetting event. On the second night, subjects thought about the humanity of the person who hurt them. They didn't diminish or excuse how they were hurt. They looked at the event differently, reflecting on how it highlighted the person's need for positive change.

This is known as compassionate reappraisal, which Charlotte vanOyen-Witvliet has been studying for several decades. I spoke with vanOyen-Witvliet about what this type of reappraisal process entails and what it aims to achieve. VanOyen-Wivliet has extensively researched the effects of holding grudges. She told me how nursing a grudge can make people feel a bit more powerful and a little less sad. Yet people's anger often persists, which can activate a stress response.

When she first started this research, vanOyen-Witvliet was asked if forgiveness is for wimps. Isn't it for the weak? She explained that it is quite the opposite. When people can forgive someone who has wronged them, their empathy and forgiveness give them a sense of control that is even greater than holding on to a grudge, she explained. Anger and sadness dissipate, sweat levels and heart rate calm down. Facial muscles relax.

She explained that ruminating over past offenses doesn't make the hurt go away. The question is, can we truly wish that good comes to the person who has hurt us? "It's not being a doormat. It's not minimizing. It's not excusing," said the psychology professor at Belmont University and an author of the study. "It's about seeing the person as a human who needs positive change and the fact that we're in a position to desire that good change for them." Forgiveness and empathy have the power to improve not only our waking well-being, but also our sleep.

On the second night of the study, after subjects thought and wrote about their offender's humanity and genuinely wished them well, the participants fell asleep faster and stayed asleep longer, with fewer disturbances. The next day, they woke up more refreshed and reported being significantly less upset by the event. Even though the situation wasn't resolved with the person who hurt them, subjects had found a kind of peace with the situation by rethinking it in a more positive and helpful way.

Ruminating about mistakes or doubts about our own lives can also keep us up at night. Perfectionism is linked to insomnia, a chronic and widespread sleep problem. Approximately 59 percent of American adults struggle to fall asleep every night or almost every night, according to a survey by the National Sleep Foundation.[26] It is common to have the occasional sleepless or restless night. Ruminating over missteps and mistakes—both real and imagined—can wreak havoc with our sleep. Thoughts of regret, shame, and guilt affect our ability to drift off. A recent study found that ruminating over negative thoughts before bed increased threatening and negative dreams.[27] How, I wondered, do we stop ruminating at night? One idea is to pick a time during the day to think through our worries so they're not as overwhelming when we try to fall asleep.

Run Away

ANOTHER DIMENSION OF DREAMING is nightmares. These are disturbing and, in some cases, trauma-related dreams that often cause the person to bolt awake, leaving the terrifying situation unresolved. Nightmares are not simply bad dreams. They can be debilitating and traumatic on their own, making nightmare sufferers terrified to fall asleep. Like recurrent dreams, there are common themes that play out across nightmares. The most common is physical aggression followed by failure or helplessness, health concerns, and worry. Dreamers report accidents, "evil forces," and being chased. In addition to fear, nightmares may express anger, sadness, and frustration.[28] Nightmares happen mostly in REM sleep, which is characterized by emotional and vivid dreams.

Approximately 5 percent of the general population have frequent nightmares, with at least one a week, while many people have the occasional nightmare. Women have more nightmares than men, and nightmares are more common among children.[29] I found that one way to understand this was to look at Tore Nielsen's Stress Acceleration Hypothesis. It is well established that a traumatic event can lead to post-traumatic nightmares. Similarly, Nielsen found that children who experience adverse events during sensitive times when they are maturing emotionally may become more susceptible to mental illness and increase their risk of nightmares over the long term.[30]

There is a strong connection between nightmares and mental health. Approximately 30 percent of people experiencing anxiety and depression suffer from nightmares.[31] One of the main symptoms of PTSD is recurrent nightmares. On their own, frequent nightmares increase the risk of suicide.[32] One study found that the frequency of disturbing dreams during early adolescence can predict suicidal ideation, which may help to identify teenagers who are at risk of suicide.[33] In another study, Zadra found that by twelve to thirteen years old, young people with suicidal ideations had more disturbing dreams compared to subjects without suicidal thoughts.[34]

Nightmare frequency is influenced by several contributing factors, including genetics, early adverse events including childhood trauma, and personality factors. Some of us are more prone to nightmares during times of stress. We experience and process stress differently. We can also be a poor judge as to whether our system is stressed out biologically, said Zadra. Biological stress markers often don't correlate with our subjective impression of stress, he explained. We might think we're not stressed, only to find out that certain stress hormones are elevated. We deal with many kinds of stress at different times, including losing a job, getting a divorce, or coping with a traumatic event.

There are two types of nightmares: idiopathic, which seem to happen without any explanation, and post-traumatic nightmares, which occur after a traumatic event. Approximately 50 percent to 70 percent of people with PTSD suffer from recurrent nightmares, which often continue for years.[35] Nightmare disorder, which is characterized by severe distress or impaired functioning, with at least one nightmare a week, often goes undiagnosed. Overall, nightmares are commonly left untreated. Often, people cope by waking themselves up or trying to push the disturbing dreams to the back of their minds. These kinds of avoidance strategies don't work in the long term.

In one of my conversations with dream researcher Michael Schredl, we talked about why such avoidance tactics are unhelpful. We looked at nightmares in relation to anxiety disorders. He gave the example of arachnophobia. If I had a fear of spiders and worked hard to avoid the little creatures that made my skin crawl, this short-term fix wouldn't solve my long-term problem. In fact, it would only make things worse. "Phobias arise because you are avoiding experiencing anxiety," said Schredl, who pointed out that the same situation would happen if I bolted awake during a nightmare. "Waking up from a dream situation is the ultimate avoidance strategy," he explained.

Rescripting Nightmares

IMAGERY REHEARSAL THERAPY (IRT), a type of cognitive behavioural therapy, is an effective treatment for nightmares. Nightmare sufferers learn to rewrite their upsetting dreams. Not only do people face their nightmares, they rescript them, which also changes people's reaction. Here's how it works. With the guidance of a mental health professional, people take the difficult first step in confronting their nightmare. They do this by recording their dream. The next step is to rewrite the nightmare. While this is up to the dreamer, a therapist helps to guide them toward an effective resolution to their disturbing scenario.

I told Schredl about my recurrent falling dream in which I woke up just before I hit the ground. I tried to think of ways that I could rescript the dream. What if I incorporated a soft mattress into my dream to cushion my fall? Or maybe I could stop myself from falling altogether? Schredl told me the mattress idea was better than if I prevented myself from falling. If I placed the mattress underneath the scaffolding, I still had the experience of falling. I didn't avoid the situation. This allowed me to change the content of the dream as well as my reaction to the situation. So if I had another falling dream in the future, I would know what to do. Typically, in a nightmare, a dreamer panics. With IRT, "the mindset is changing," said Schredl. This equips the person with a new thought pattern that can lead them to a solution. The problem-solving aspect of IRT puts the dreamer in control.

In the next step of IRT, a dreamer writes down their new version of the nightmare. The process can be adapted for children who use drawings to reimagine their terrifying dreams. Then every day for two weeks, the person takes a few minutes to imagine their rewritten nightmare. So when they have the terrifying dream again, they no longer watch helplessly as events unfold. They can save themselves from their nightmare scenario.

In speaking with Zadra, I learned that rewriting a nightmare is not necessarily about changing the ending. It's about rescripting what feels right for the person, he explained. Some people might find relief in changing minor details. Zadra gave the example of a woman who altered the colour of the walls in her nightmare.

I kept thinking about my falling dream. I had to ask Schredl what the recurrent dream might be about. "Dreams are exaggerations of waking life feelings," he said. A falling dream "is the most potent or most graphic way to depict the feeling of helplessness." It was always the same. I found myself free-falling through darkness, and I knew that if I hit the ground, I would die. My dream-self was convinced of it. "So that's a pure feeling of helplessness," said Schredl, who explained that people may feel helpless for many reasons. Maybe they were looking for a job or there was uncertainty in a relationship. I decided I would start tracking when I had my falling dream and connect it with what was happening in my life.

While IRT is very effective, the technique is relatively unknown and underutilized by clinicians. Only one-third of frequent nightmare sufferers seek help, and many who do reach out for professional support find it unhelpful. In one study, only 33 percent of people thought there was a cure for nightmares.[36] Some people cope by sharing their disturbing dreams with family or friends. Dream sharing can give an immediate feeling of relief. It might convince people that they can move on and forget about their nightmare. But the effect doesn't usually last. Facing a disturbing nightmare is only part of the solution. I learned that the problem-solving aspect of IRT is what makes it so effective. Remarkably, it can take less than an hour for nightmare sufferers to find some relief.

In a recent study, Schredl gave subjects a single thirty-minute IRT session. In the short phone session, people shared their nightmares and devised ways to rescript them. If they used avoidance behaviour like my idea to prevent myself from falling, subjects were guided toward more solution-based actions. For two weeks after the phone session, subjects practiced their rescripted nightmares. After the short-term IRT, 78 percent of participants reported little or no nightmare distress.

The study showed that a brief IRT session can reduce nightmares and their associated distress. For nightmare sufferers, "you know you can do something. Self-sufficiency," said Schredl. "You have a new skill where you can confront and remodel your anxieties that occurred in the dream."

There is another novel treatment for nightmares that is currently being investigated, which focuses on creating an experience of control. Dream researcher Adam Haar told me about his recent pilot study with Westley Youngren that explored how dreaming can be used as a therapeutic tool to reduce nightmares and traumatic dreams. Research shows that frequent nightmares increase the risk of suicide. Constant nightmares often lead to feelings of helplessness. Many people believe there is nothing they can do to stop their distressing and often debilitating dreams. One way to lower suicidal thoughts is to help people feel more in control of their lives, and an innovative way to achieve this is through their dreams.

The researchers gathered fifteen nightmare sufferers and trained them on a technique called Targeted Dream Incubation (TDI) that uses simple prompts to help them guide their dream thoughts. During the first few minutes of sleep, a recording instructed the participants, "while you try to fall asleep, try and think of a tree." Then they were left to nap for ninety minutes. People were assessed once they awoke and a week later. The researchers found a significant reduction in suicidal thoughts after using TDI, and this positive effect contin-ued a week later.[37] "By helping people feel more in control, you can see their ideation around suicide is lower because they're less afraid of sleeping and per-haps sleep better because of it," said Haar. People learn that they don't have to accept their nightmares. There is in fact a way out of their distressing dreams.

With TDI, people have "a concrete experience of control" as they guide their dreams, said Haar. People learn and remember through an empowering experi-ence. This sense of control is key to helping people overcome their nightmares. If they are able to control their dreams, even in a small way, they're more likely to believe they can control their nightmares. This gives people the motivation to stay in treatment and have better outcomes, explained Haar. These different techniques offer hope to the numerous people with debilitating nightmares.

This idea led me to the last point I wanted to explore in relation to dreams and well-being. Why can it seem impossible to hide from our preoccupa-tions and fears, even in our dreams? This question led me to the white bear experiment.

Can't Get You Out of My Head

DURING THE COVID-19 PANDEMIC, many of us discovered that hushing our anx-ious thoughts during the day made them scream for our attention at night. It was as if the act of avoiding these unwanted thoughts brought them back with a vengeance when our defenses were down and we drifted off to sleep. This is the power of suppression. Scientists have discovered that if you spend your day trying to avoid a certain thought, a part of your mind is constantly searching for that unwanted thought. This cognitive hide-and-seek continues when you lie down at night, and the uninvited thought might show up in your dreams.

To understand the mental mechanics of suppression, I began by looking at what a suppressed thought is and how it is formed in the mind. Suppressed thoughts are different than repressed thoughts, which Freud was famous for interpreting in dreams. Repression is the involuntary act of forgetting. It happens in the realm of our unconscious. I could be typing this sentence and not realize that I am inadvertently repressing another thought. Freud would use a hidden wish or desire as an example. But repressed thoughts can also be neutral.

Suppression is the flip side of repression. It's the conscious and deliberate act of doing everything in your power to forget. To test this out, I let my mind sift through its catalogue of memories until it found something I didn't want to think about. A few days before, I had foolishly tried to cut a partially frozen bagel. The knife skated off the hard bagel and into my palm, causing a deep cut. Oh, how I wanted to forget that memory. It was taking up too much mental real estate. But I let it play out again in my mind and took some time to think about it. Then after a few minutes, I tried to push away the thought. It wasn't so easy. I could distract myself for a few moments while I focused on returning some emails. But the thought kept popping back into my head when I least expected it.

Thought suppression isn't always a bad thing. In fact, it's important to be able to control our thoughts at certain times. There are many different reasons and motivations for suppression. It could be an emotional thought that causes pain and upset, which could range from everyday troubles to ongoing struggles with depression, addiction, and past trauma. Maybe it's an attempt at self-control, like trying to forget about the bag of chips in the cupboard. Or maybe there is a need to keep a secret, like when I ran into a friend and stopped myself from blurting out that I would see them at their surprise birthday party.

Yet motivation is irrelevant to the act of suppression. "Once you start that process, then it starts popping back to mind just because of suppression. So you can end up thinking it's far more important, far more central, far more deep and revealing about who you are simply because you can't get rid of it anymore," explained the late Daniel M. Wegner when I spoke with him some years ago. This made me think of a song that gets stuck in your head. While it's possible that the song may have personal significance, it could also be stuck on repeat simply because you want to forget about it. It's the act of trying to suppress those catchy tunes that causes them to play on an endless loop in your head.

During his decades of study on thought suppression, Wegner came up with the ironic process theory to explain what is happening in the mind when we try to forget about something. There are two mental processes going on as we try to control what we're thinking. There is the conscious and deliberate operating process that searches for distractions to keep our mind busy and away from an unwanted thought. At the same time, the unconscious and involuntary ironic process acts as a hall monitor walking the corridors of our mind, searching for the unwanted thought. When things go according to plan, both mental processes work together to achieve suppression.

But this can only go on for so long. "You've set that little ticking bomb," Wegner explained. A part of your unconscious mind searches for the "failure" of your mental control. "That part of your mind actually then produces the failure." Then the suppressed thought barges in. The harder we try to avoid thinking about something, the more likely that pesky thought will return uninvited. "If you spend your whole day trying not to think about something, you really do get a part of your mind looking for it all the time," said Wegner.

Wegner tested this theory with his famous "white bear" experiment. The Harvard scientist was inspired by Russian author Fyodor Dostoyevsky's comment in "Winter Notes on Summer Impression." Dostoyevsky wrote, "Try to pose for yourself this task: not to think of a polar bear, and you will see that the cursed thing will come to mind every minute." A white bear doesn't conjure strong emotions for most people. It made me wonder, is it really that hard to suppress such a neutral thought?

Wegner and his team devised a simple experiment to test Dostoyevsky's idea. They instructed subjects to suppress the thought of a white bear. Then each subject was asked to talk about whatever came to mind, ringing a bell every time they thought of a white bear. Participants rang the bell more than once a minute on average. Then the researchers switched things around. This time, they asked the subjects to focus on a white bear. When they were asked to talk about whatever came to mind, the subjects thought of a white bear even more than another group that had been asked to think of the white bear from the start. The experiment showed that the initial thought suppression caused a greater "rebound" of the white bear in people's minds compared to those who were free to think of the white bear the entire time. Then many years later, Wegner tested the power of thought suppression on dreams.

In 2001, Megan Kozak Williams, a young graduate student from New Jersey, was faced with the daunting task of picking a first-year project for her PhD in social psychology. Wegner was her mentor at Harvard, and the pair began discussing possible topics of study. Kozak Williams was interested in states of consciousness. "We all have these inner worlds going on that no one is privy to, and I think that dreams are an example of that," said Kozak Williams, who is now an associate professor of psychology at Oregon's Linfield University. She and Wegner started to think about thought suppression in relation to the dreaming mind. Would it be possible to get the same rebound effect in dreams that Wegner had found in waking life?

To test this idea, Wegner and Kozak Williams teamed up with Richard M. Wenzlaff and devised a simple at-home experiment. They gathered psychology students from the University of Texas in San Antonio and separated them into three groups: suppression, expression, and mention. For the experiment, subjects followed their usual bedtime routine. But before falling asleep, they opened a sealed envelope to find simple instructions: think of a "crush," someone they were emotionally attracted to, and also a "non-crush" they knew but had no emotional attraction to.

The "suppression" group was instructed to think of anything except the target person, either their crush or their non-crush, for five minutes. The "expression" group was told to focus on their target person, and the "mention" group was to provide the initials of their target person before thinking about anything. All subjects were asked to write stream-of-consciousness thoughts for five minutes, and indicate with a checkmark every time they thought of their target person. Everyone then went to sleep as usual. In the morning, participants recorded their dreams and noted how often their target person appeared.

Students who tried to avoid thinking of a specific person were more likely to dream of this person than students who thought about their target individual or provided the target person's initials before sleep. Interestingly, this was true for both a crush and a non-crush.

The study showed that if we try to avoid thinking about someone, there is a good chance they will show up in our dreams, regardless of our attraction to the person. The experiment suggested that the act of suppression makes a thought rebound in our dreams, not our feelings for someone. The researchers concluded that suppressed thoughts rebound whether we wish for these thoughts or not.[38] Another remarkable aspect was the time lapse between the suppressed thought and when it showed up much later in people's dreams.

In a later study, Wegner discovered that stress has an impact on suppression. I thought that stress would take our mind off a suppressed thought. But in fact Wegner found the opposite. He discovered that stress eroded the mental process that we employ to distract ourselves. When I asked him how this works, Wegner gave the example of trying to forget about a white bear while remembering a ten-digit number. This mental juggle would result in more white bear thoughts. The additional mental load would make it even more difficult to forget about the bear.

"You'd think stress would take your mind off things because you're paying attention to the stress," he told me. "But in fact it destroys that process you're using to distract yourself." How could I apply this knowledge to my everyday life? "You're going to be successful if you can manage to suppress thoughts without being under stress," he explained. "When you are given plenty of time to get yourself away from the thought."

What do we do if we can't suppress distressing thoughts? Wegner was asked this often. He offered a few different strategies to combat our own white bear thoughts. Getting involved with important plans can create some mental distance from unwanted thoughts. It can help to dedicate a set time during the day to address concerns. When unwanted thoughts appear, we can tell ourselves it's not the right time to think about them. Reducing multi-tasking can ease our mental load, which makes thought suppression even more difficult. Meditation and mindfulness work on mental control, which may help deflect unwanted thoughts.[39]

Research has shown the powerful connection between dreams and well-being. If we're in a positive state of mind, there is a chance that we will have positive dreams. The downside is that low levels of well-being often lead to bad dreams. While it's difficult to face our fears and battle personal conflicts during sleep, it's not necessarily a bad thing. Emotional and threatening dreams can prepare us for life's dangers, in their many guises.

Chapter Five

The Safe Space
of Dreams

WHEN ROSALIND CARTWRIGHT WAS IN HER LATE THIRTIES, HER husband walked out, leaving Cartwright with two young daughters and many sleepless nights. When she did manage to sleep, Cartwright's dreams were fueled with anxiety. She decided to stop all the tossing and turning and put her endless nights to good use. Cartwright hired a babysitter to look after her girls and launched a sleep laboratory at the University of Illinois, where she taught psychology.

The late pioneering dream researcher didn't start out in sleep. In the early 1940s, she trained as a research psychologist at the University of Toronto, and continued her education at Cornell later that decade. From there, she worked at the University of Chicago, for psychotherapist Carl Rogers, who used psychotherapy to get patients to acknowledge their innermost feelings as aspects of their personal identities. Together, Cartwright and Rogers explored ways people could work through their fear and depression to move on with life. Cartwright worked next door to Nathaniel Kleitman, who at the time was researching the parameters of sleep with Eugene Aserinsky and William Dement. Cartwright learned everything she could about the field. She approached Allan Rechtschaffen, a friend and influential sleep researcher, who taught her how to set up and wire a lab.

Then in the early 1960s, while going through her divorce, Cartwright constructed a sleep lab at the University of Illinois College of Medicine. She converted a men's bathroom in an empty psychiatric unit at the medical college, replacing tubs with beds and installing foam tiles to help with acoustics. It turned out that subjects couldn't sleep in the soundproof space. So Cartwright let in some noise from the street.[1]

In the stillness of the lab, Cartwright experienced a connection with her mother, Stella (Hein) Falk, a poet who found creative inspiration in the images of her rich dream life. When Falk shared her dream stories at the dinner table, Cartwright's father, Henry Falk, would say, "Stella, you have such an interesting night life."[2] Cartwright's mother also felt that sleep had healing qualities. Growing up, Cartwright and her siblings referred to their home as "the house of sacred sleep." Alone in the lab, Cartwright discovered what would become her lifelong mission: to study the valuable resource of dreams, especially during times of personal crisis.

Cartwright discovered that for many people, it was a difficult and slow process to recognize and accept the emotions that were holding them back. Yet they could identify their worries and uncertainties when these played out in their dreams. People's dream life offered a window into waking life.

During the day, we might fool ourselves and others about how we are feeling. Our dreams often tell a different story. Psychologically, we live in two different worlds, explained Cartwright. In dreams, "we bare our private biases, perceptions, and motivations."[3] We connect past experiences and thoughts to our present circumstances, providing new perspectives. Dreams also reveal how we cope when things get tough, said Cartwright. Do we run from danger? Or do we face our fears? Dreams offer a safe space to play out our darkest fears.

Cartwright set out to investigate whether dreams could help us heal, especially when faced with a personal crisis, and how to fix our dreams when they get stuck or malfunction. Our sense of self can become shaky when we lose someone close to us, our marriage dissolves, or we are let go from a job. Loss and uncertainty can impact our dreams. When I read about Cartwright's work, it made me wonder why some of us take longer than others to recover from life's blows. Did it have anything to do with our dream life? Could we use our dreams to speed up the recovery process?

Cartwright discovered that divorce was an ideal model to study the function of dreams during times of personal stress and upheaval. It was the late 1970s, and divorce had become a widespread problem, challenging people to question their changing roles. Divorce can involve competing and shifting feelings of anger, guilt, and regret as people struggle with their sense of self. Also, divorce has many commonalities with some of life's other traumas. As she saw it, the loss of a marriage can be as wrenching as the death of a loved one, and those going through divorce often blamed themselves, which survivors of assault may also experience.

Cartwright posted ads in local newspapers, offering a small fee to spend three nights in the sleep lab. She gathered seventy participants going through a divorce. It had to be their first marriage that had to have lasted at least three years. Thirty of the participants were doing well, while forty found it difficult to cope with their divorce. Both groups had the same number of men and women. Most subjects were in their mid-thirties with children. The participants were diverse in race, occupation, income level, and education. There was an equal number of partners who had left their spouses and those whose spouses had left them.

Some people came for the small remuneration. Others wanted to know more about dreams. The majority wanted to talk about their failed marriage and try to make sense of it. Cartwright interviewed subjects about their marriage, how it started, developed, and dissolved.

During the first two nights, subjects became comfortable with the lab environment. On night three, they were awoken in each successive period of REM sleep to report what was going through their minds. The following morning, Cartwright spoke with them, looking for possible connections between dreams and learn how they were coping.

A year later, Cartwright discovered that some people were coping far better than others. Remarkably, those who had dreamt about the pain of their divorce had recovered from their personal crisis and no longer struggled with depression. The subjects who didn't dream about the upset of their divorce remained stuck in their distressing situation and continued to battle symptoms of depression. "A bad dream, like an elevated temperature, is a symptom that something is wrong," explained Cartwright. "It is a distress signal, a message from our sleeping mind to our waking mind that is risky to ignore."

In speaking with participants, Cartwright discovered that dreams helped people review and revise their sense of self and rehearse new possibilities for the future. She found that if dreams function properly, they also help to repair what is stuck within us. In dreams, we are able to put things in perspective and think creatively about what is troubling us.

Cartwright developed the Crisis Dreaming Method to help people recast dreams that contribute to a poor self-image. Through this approach, people identify their current issues, then remember times they felt happy and strong. People are encouraged to question why particular dreams show up at certain times. To answer this, they reflect on the themes that link dreams to waking life. This helps people improve their outlook in waking life and prepare for future problems.

Cartwright explained why some of us have an easier time navigating life's rough patches. If we have long-time friends, they can help us remember who we are, because they expect us to hold a constant place in their lives. We remain stable around them, and in character. Our genetic makeup can affect the way we deal with stress. A healthy self-image helps us cope with problems without blaming ourselves, and we can seek help when we need it. It's also important to use our dreams to improve our waking lives.

Dreams highlight rather than erase experience, "to help us maintain and update our internal emotional picture of ourselves," noted Cartwright.[4] The emotional processing of dreams helps us preserve our sense of self as our place in the world changes.

Boundaries of the Dreaming Mind

DREAMING IS OUR PRIVATE nightly therapy session, said American sleep researcher and psychoanalyst Ernest Hartmann. The idea of psychotherapy is to make free associations, which puts you in a dreamlike state, explained the late Hartmann when we spoke some years ago. Maybe dreaming functions in a therapy-like way, he said, making new connections with old memories and integrating new material into old pathways. Our waking and dreaming thoughts are on the same continuum. We are the same person when we dream. Yet we are able to think more loosely, just like in therapy.

We don't need to remember our dreams to gain their therapeutic benefit. But if we do remember them, they offer an additional function, letting us use our dreams consciously, on our own or in therapy. By reflecting on our dreams, we are given new perspectives on ourselves and the thoughts that preoccupy us. Dreams open our eyes to a new way of seeing.

During his many years as a psychotherapist, Hartmann observed that after a traumatic event, pieces of the event played out in people's dreams. As time went on, dreams often pictured the person's dominant emotions. Often, there were many emotions wrapped up in a dream. When there was one overpowering emotion, Hartmann found that it created a central image. Tidal wave dreams often happened after a traumatic event, including a terrible accident, a natural disaster, or an attack.

During one of our discussions, Hartmann explained that a central image wasn't necessarily an accurate representation of the traumatic event. It was more about the central emotion. He offered the example of a man who survived a house fire. The man didn't live near water and hadn't been to the ocean for more than a year. Yet he dreamt of being swept away by a massive tidal wave and struggled to come to the surface as he awoke. The man felt vulnerable, and the central image of the tidal wave pictured this overwhelming emotion. After a traumatic event, the intensity of a dream's central image is high, said Hartmann, which mirrors the intensity of the dreamer's emotions.[5]

Hartmann found that after a traumatic event, people sometimes connected the present trauma with past traumas or experiences that had an emotional connection. This helped them realize that the current trauma might not be the most distressing thing to ever happen. It also diminished the distress of a future traumatic event as the person had already worked through something similar in their mind. Later on, a person's dream life picked up its usual themes that had nothing to do with the traumatic event. Maybe they resumed dreaming about work or a relationship.

The 9/11 terrorist attacks provided an opportunity to study dreams before and after a traumatic event that had an impact on people's psychological well-being. In one study, Hartmann examined the dreams of forty-four people living across the United States. None of the participants resided in Manhattan or lost any relatives or close friends to the terrorist attacks. The participants had recorded their dreams for several years. Each participant sent Hartmann twenty dreams—the last 10 dreams recorded before the terrorist attacks and the 10 dreams after 9/11. This provided more than 880 dreams for Hartmann to analyze.

The results were remarkably clear-cut. While all the participants had watched replays of the events of 9/11 on TV, they didn't dream about tall buildings or planes more frequently. The outstanding feature was the emotional intensity reflected in people's dreams. There was a significant increase in the intensity of the central image. When it came to the dominant emotion across dreams, Hartmann found a strong trend toward more fear/terror in the aftermath of 9/11. The results showed that the dreams after 9/11 didn't change because of exposure to images of the terrorist attack. It was the emotions evoked by the event that changed people's dreams. Hartmann pointed out that the planes crashing into the Twin Towers had become a tidal wave that appeared in people's dreams during the time of emotional stress. The study also reflected Hartmann's concept that dreams are new creations guided by a dreamer's emotions rather than replays of waking events.[6]

A dream, like a work of art, compiles old material to create something novel and unique. A dreamer, like an artist, is guided by their emotions. Just as each of us thinks differently, we dream differently. In speaking with Hartmann, I learned how personality plays a role. Specifically, a dimension of personality that Hartmann called "boundaries of the mind," internal barriers that determine whether we can get in touch with our dreams. Hartmann believed that everything our mind houses—our emotions, thoughts, and memories—is separated as well as connected by boundaries. These boundaries can be thick or thin, depending on our personality.

Some people are resistant to emotion. They are pragmatic and rational, living orderly lives. Hartmann saw them as having thick boundaries. On the other end, there are those who openly express their feelings and tend to be vulnerable and sensitive. Hartmann imagined these individuals had thin boundaries. Most people aren't one extreme or the other but rather fall somewhere in between.

By examining boundaries of personality, Hartmann believed, we can understand aspects of ourselves that are often overlooked. We have boundaries of emotion, which determine whether we are in touch with our feelings. There are boundaries of memory that explain how we sort and call upon recollections from the recent and distant past. There are boundaries around our identity, which is either fluid or fixed. Then there are the boundaries between sleep and waking life.

Hartmann discovered that most people with thick boundaries easily separated their waking from their dreaming lives. They had a sharp focus of thought, concentrating on one thing at a time. They didn't let their emotions cloud their thinking. Often, they didn't recall their dreams as easily as those with thin boundaries. By contrast, people with thin boundaries had more emotionally charged dreams. Their dream life seeped into their waking existence, where they often spent time daydreaming.

To understand how personality affected dreams, Hartmann decided to study an emotional and intense type of dream: the nightmare. Why are some of us tormented by nightmares while others slumber in peace? Intent to find out, Hartmann recruited fifty volunteers between the ages of twenty and fifty who had chronic nightmares.[7] The similarities Hartmann found among his subjects were fascinating. Most were in the arts, and included musicians, music teachers, and art therapists. Subjects were emotional and open with their thoughts and feelings, revealing intimate details about their lives. They tended to form romantic attachments quickly, sometimes developing unhealthy relationships. Yet they weren't afraid to walk alone at night in dangerous neighbourhoods. Many were easily taken for granted and experienced everyday pitfalls as intense blows.

Reflecting on the common characteristics of subjects—their sensitivity, unguarded natures, and susceptibility to their emotions—Hartmann concluded that the nightmare sufferers had thin boundaries of personality. They didn't compartmentalize the world with barriers. They often found it hard to wake up, even questioning whether they were awake after intense dreams. To test his boundaries-of-personality theory among the general population, Hartmann created the Boundary Questionnaire. It looked at many kinds of boundaries in people's lives, including ones they maintained between themselves and others and internal boundaries between themselves and their innermost feelings.

Of the more than one thousand people who took the questionnaire, Hartmann found those with thin boundaries had the best dream recall. When I thought about it, this made sense. When we remember a dream, we are in a sense crossing a boundary by recollecting something that happened in sleep. The thin boundary group had dreams that were more vivid, emotional, and bizarre. Many from the thick boundary group said they were distant and unengaged with their dreams.

During the day, we often think along straight lines or fall into ruts, almost as if we are in a ditch along the side of a road, Hartmann told me. In dreams, we escape this metaphorical ditch as we think creatively and make new connections. Imagine someone was trying to decide on a career path. During the day, they might make lists of their likes and dislikes or take aptitude tests to understand their strengths. This would give them only one possible line of thinking. In many non-Western cultures, people often look to their dreams for answers. "Why not make use of our dreams?" Hartmann said. "It's another part of us. It's still ourselves. It's still our own minds, but we're functioning differently. We're seeing more broadly and widely."[8]

During our last conversation, Hartmann shared a dream that he reflected on for decades. He found himself walking along a beach. In front of him, a towering cliff rose up out of the ocean where no cliff had any right to be, he said. At the time we talked, Hartmann still questioned the possible meaning of the dream. He believed it might have been trying to explore important issues like death. Yet instead of a frightening vision of death, Hartmann saw it as a grand, impressive one. The powerful image evoked a feeling of positivity. Usually, dreams don't stay with us because of an intricate plot or fascinating character development, he explained. A dream's powerful image keeps it fresh in our mind for days, months, or even years.

Midnight Therapy Session

IN RECENT YEARS, STUDIES have examined the brain activity associated with emotional processing in sleep and dreams. There is evidence that sleep helps us process our waking stresses and emotions, and that sleep is integral to our mental health and well-being. Even the occasional sleepless night can make it difficult to weather the daily storm of hassles and worries. Sleep deprivation as well as fragmented sleep are symptoms as well as risk factors for mental health conditions including anxiety and depression.

One way to understand this is to look at sleep's important role in regulating our "emotional brain-state."[9] Studies have shown that sleep loss not only heightened negative emotions, it diminished positive feelings after people had achieved a goal, something that would normally make them feel good.[10] So how does this work? I took another look at what happens in the brain during sleep.

Brain imaging studies indicated that some brain regions associated with emotions and memory are a flurry of activity during REM sleep. This includes the brain's limbic system, which helps process and regulate emotions. At the same time, there is a reduction in noradrenaline, a chemical that's famous for our fight-or-flight response in fearful situations. Author and sleep scientist Matthew Walker questioned whether we are reprocessing emotional memories in this ideal brain state during REM sleep. Is dreaming during REM a "perfectly designed nocturnal soothing balm—one that removes the emotional sharp edges of our daily lives?" asked Walker in *Why We Sleep: Unlocking the Power of Sleep and Dreams*.[11] But how exactly do we reprocess and consolidate emotional memories?

As I worked my way through many of Walker's studies on dreams, emotions, and memory, I found the well-known model of dreams as overnight therapy. In a 2009 study, Walker and Els van der Helm put forth their Sleep to Forget and Sleep to Remember hypothesis. Emotionally charged experiences tend to create emotional memories. Yet when we recall these memories later on, we might not have the same emotional reaction as we had to the original experience. The idea is, the overnight therapy of REM sleep has removed the "bitter emotional rind from the information-rich fruit," explained Walker in *Why We Sleep*. This lets us revisit emotional memories without having to relive the upsetting associated feelings in the same way. This process isn't accomplished when someone is suffering from PTSD, a severe stress response to a traumatic event that causes them to re-experience the past trauma.

According to Walker and van der Helm, we sleep to forget the emotional tone of a memory while we sleep to remember the details of important and salient experiences, weaving them into our personal library of existing knowledge. REM sleep offers an "optimal biological theatre" to make this "therapy" possible.[12]

In *Why We Sleep*, Walker described how they tested the role of sleep in emotional processing. Healthy, young participants were randomly assigned into two groups. All of the subjects looked at emotionally charged pictures while they were in an MRI machine that produced images of their brain activity. They were asked to rate their emotions. After twelve hours, the participants once again lay down in the MRI scanner to view the same emotional pictures while their brain activity was measured. Again, participants were asked to rate their level of emotions in relation to the pictures. One group of subjects saw the images in the morning and evening without any nap in between. Another group viewed the emotional images in the evening and slept through the night before seeing the images again in the morning.

Those whose sessions were interrupted by a night's sleep had a significant reduction in their emotional response to the images when they viewed them a second time. The MRI results indicated a significant decrease in amygdala reactivity during the second viewing of images. At the same time, there was reactivity in the prefrontal cortex. The subjects who didn't sleep between sessions still had a negative emotional reaction to the images when they viewed them a second time and described strong, painful feelings. The time in REM sleep gave participants "emotional convalescence," explained Walker. "To sleep, perchance to heal."[13]

Researchers continue to investigate the role of REM sleep as well as other sleep stages in emotional processing. This includes a growing interest in studying how NREM, including slow-wave sleep, might help with fear extinction and processing emotional memories.

A Little Help from Our Friends

HOW WE PROCESS EMOTIONS in our dreams could very well depend on where we call home. A recent study found that the emotional function of dreaming varies across diverse societies and provided a rare glimpse of how culture and environment shape our dreams.

The majority of dream research is conducted in Western society, mostly in the United States and Europe. In speaking with evolutionary anthropologist David R. Samson, I learned that this is problematic for many reasons. Data from Western, educated, industrialized nations are not representative of our species, said Samson, director of the Sleep and Human Evolution Lab at the University of Toronto, where he is an associate professor of evolutionary anthropology. For 99.9 percent of the human story, people lived in bands, camps, and tribes.

Today, forager communities face challenges similar to our paleolithic ancestors. They have 24/7 exposure to natural light and natural temperature variation. There is the ecological stress of the rainy versus the dry season. They're dependent on a completely different economy than Western societies. "Their economy is calories," said Samson. The most important social unit of forager groups is the camp, which is composed of twenty-five to thirty-five adults and has a strong division of labour that is based on biological sex. This living structure shapes the waking and dreaming lives of communities like the Hadza in Tanzania and the BaYaka in the Republic of the Congo.

In 2016, Samson lived with the Hadza for about three months. The Hadza live in four-by-six huts that are built by women in about four hours. If one of the women's husbands is an accomplished hunter, they might have a zebra hide on the top of the hut to offer protection during the heavy rains.

The Hadza believe that dreams have immense spiritual power. In fact, they consider it completely acceptable to adjust your waking life because of a dream. Samson spent a lot of time speaking with elders about their thoughts on the functions and uses of dreams. One elder shared a dream in which a hunting cat got him while he was scavenging a kill. After the dream, the man didn't go into the bush for three days, said Samson. I found it hard to imagine that a threatening dream could be a valid excuse to miss work in Western culture.

A few years ago, Samson, University of Geneva psychiatrist and researcher Lampros Perogamvros, and an international group of researchers set out to test whether the dreams of forager groups regulated emotions more effectively than the dreams of Western populations. They compared the dreams of Hadza and BaYaka forager communities to dreams of subjects in North America and Europe. The Global North group included young, healthy participants, people with social anxiety, and those who experienced nightmares. This totaled 234 subjects, who provided 896 dreams.

The Hadza and BaYaka reported more threats in their dreams. I could see how this made sense, considering the different kinds of threats they faced in waking life, from high infant and adolescent mortality to hunting and competition from other local tribes. The results took an interesting turn when the researchers measured the emotional effect of the forager groups' dreams. When faced with threats in day-to-day life, the dreamers weren't overly distressed. They had low levels of anxiety and negative emotions compared to Western subjects with social anxiety or nightmares as well as healthy Western participants. The nightmare group reported significantly more negative emotions despite having fewer threats in their dreams. I found it fascinating. The study showed that the forager communities were regulating their emotions in their dreams.

How did they do it? One aspect stood out: they weren't alone. The forager groups overcame danger or survived life-threatening situations in their dreams with the help of their community. One Hadza dreamt he fell into a well, and his friend helped him get out. Another Hadza dreamt he was hit by a buffalo in the bushland where the group looks for honey. A man named January helped him.[14] Their dreams expressed their socially connected and dependent way of life.

This was in stark contrast to the dreams of the Global North subjects, who found themselves mostly alone. Samson pointed to the epidemic of isolation and loneliness in Western society. "We don't have the strong social ties embedded into not only our physical space, but also our psychic space, that help us overcome these challenges," he said.

When the forager groups were faced with threats in their dreams, they came up with adaptive responses to them, offering a cathartic experience that was beneficial for the dreamer. "It's like a heathy cognitive immune system working through challenges," said Samson, "and it seems like that's the thing that we probably all wish we had." It's emotional catharsis and fear extinction all in one, helping people regulate their emotions and mentally prepare for whatever challenges life may serve.

Samson and I talked about the importance of paying attention to our dreams and what they might be trying to tell us. "Even in our socially atrophied Western context," said Samson, "there is an adaptive component. Something that can enhance the likelihood of survival reproduction."

We bias awake as being the crucial element to natural selection, said Samson. "The beauty to me, the sort of poetry of all this, is we can see natural selection perhaps shaping alternate states of consciousness for life on this earth," he said. We talked about how there has to be a good reason why we would shut down and sleep at night, making ourselves vulnerable to a potentially vicious environment. "The juice has to be worth the evolutionary squeeze," he said. "I think there's some evidence supporting this idea that even in altered states of consciousness, evolution is still working."

This reminded me of the Threat Simulation Theory, an evolutionary theory on the function of dreaming. Could dreams act as threat rehearsals for the pitfalls and troubles of everyday life?

Fight, Run, Repeat

AS A CHILD, FINNISH cognitive neuroscientist Antti Revonsuo spent his summers in a log cabin overlooking the sea. An hour's drive from Turku, Finland, it was a rugged and remote place from another time. His family's cabin was on the same land as his grandparents' farmhouse, which was built without electricity or running water. There was an old cattle house and sauna. The buildings were nestled among fields and forests, and there wasn't another house in sight. There were intense summer storms, and Revonsuo watched ominous clouds gather on the horizon and roll across the water toward his cabin.

Sometimes a storm would come in the middle of the night, with the loud rumble of thunderclouds and flashes of lightning across the sea. His parents would waken him and they'd run to the safety of their car to wait out the storm. These were terrifying experiences that stayed with Revonsuo, finding their way into his dreams for decades. During his PhD thesis, he had recurrent dreams of trying to escape an incoming storm. Sometimes he'd combine his childhood memory with another imagined threat that was visually similar. The flash and rumble of his storm dreams would get mixed up with the pressure wave of a nuclear explosion from *Terminator 2*, leaving him to wonder what he was running from.

For his PhD on consciousness, Revonsuo wanted to study dreaming. It was the mid-1990s and there weren't any supervisors who specialized in this altered state of consciousness. So he and some classmates started their own dream group, recording their dreams and reading the existing literature. They questioned the phenomenon of dreaming, exploring how the dreaming brain creates an entire world of consciousness that is eerily similar to the external world. Revonsuo came across the work of David Foulkes, who characterized dreams as "credible world analogs" and "simulations" of waking experience.[15] Building on this idea, Revonsuo saw dreaming as a natural virtual reality constructed by the brain. He applied the same idea to waking consciousness.

During one of our conversations, Revonsuo told me how it works. When we are awake, this virtual reality is online with our sensory mechanisms constantly feeding our brain information. Everything around us seems to be outside of ourselves. The keyboard that I'm typing on, the window that I look out as I pause to think of this sentence, all these objects are outside of myself. But the experience of hitting the keys or looking at the trees swaying in the breeze is happening in my brain. This is the same system that creates dream experiences. The illusion that we are in direct contact with a physical world that is outside of our body and our brain is what's known in philosophy as naïve realism. But it's happening in the brain, just like in dreaming. This virtual reality is more convincing when we're dreaming and out of touch with the outside world. "During wakefulness, we fall for this naïve realism," Revonsuo told me. "We think that when we look around, we actually see a real world that is independent of ourselves. But it's also a kind of dream world." We get tricked because our brain "is getting constant input that stays much more stable and coheres with what is actually out there."

Revonsuo began to wonder why the dreaming brain would construct such a complicated state of consciousness at a time when we can't interact with the world. Why would the brain use so much energy to construct this virtual reality experience? He thought of complex flight simulators that are used to train pilots. A simulator allows pilots to experience everyday and rare or exaggerated situations. Imagine the day these trained pilots faced a similar threat. They would be prepared and know exactly what to do. The learning is all there in the brain, said Revonsuo. Even though the training is a simulation, the experience feels so real that the learning effect ensures "you won't panic. You will go into this track where you were in the simulation," he said. "So that you stay cool and you just act." A key element to the simulated training is the variability. By testing out various combinations of different threats and environments, pilots figure out the best way to handle a situation. He thought that the same learning seems to happen in dreams.

In dreams, we create all kinds of threatening situations to test out. We might search frantically for a lost child or fight an invisible virus. In one study of healthy adults, Revonsuo found that 60 percent to 75 percent of dream reports contained at least one threatening event. Somehow, the mechanism that produces dreams has an internal bias that exaggerates the number of dangerous events that we encounter, said Revonsuo. It doesn't replicate real life. "The dream world is a much more dangerous or risky place than the waking world," he warned. Just like the unpredictable virtual world of a flight simulator.

Revonsuo asked me to imagine if pilots performed an eight-hour flight simulation, and nothing happened. "That's not really training anything except boredom," he said. The real learning would come when pilots faced unexpected problems. "And that's exactly how our dream production mechanism seems to be preprogrammed," he said. "So that it exaggerates negative and potentially harmful events."

In 2000, Revonsuo published his Threat Simulation Theory (TST). He proposed that the biological function of dreaming is to simulate threatening situations in order to rehearse and prepare for life's dangers. This dates back to the hunter-gatherers of the prehistoric Pleistocene era, who were in a constant fight for survival.This fight-or-flight situation continued for hundreds of thousands of years. Revonsuo's idea is that the dreaming brain was evolving at the same time, developing an adaptive function to help us prepare for potential risks. Revonsuo isn't saying that all dreams have this adaptive function. The threat-simulation system kicks in when we need to rehearse skills for survival.[16] This depends on what is happening around us.

To test whether early exposure to real threats activates the threat-simulation system, Revonsuo analyzed the dreams of three groups of children from Finland and Iraq. The Finnish children lived in a safe environment. Two groups of Kurdish children lived with the constant threat of danger in northern Iraq, where Kurdish people were persecuted by the Iraqi military. Only one group of Kurdish children had experienced a personal trauma, including witnessing a killing, losing a loved one, or having their home destroyed.

All of the children dreamt of similar types of threatening events. They dreamt of accidents and narrow escapes from danger, illnesses, and aggressive encounters. The big difference was the frequency and severity of these threats. The Kurdish children who had experienced trauma during the day faced more threats in their dreams. Almost 80 percent of their dreams had at least one threatening event compared to 56 percent of the dreams of the Kurdish children who hadn't personally experienced trauma. In comparison, 31 percent of the Finnish children's dreams contained a threatening event.[17] While Finnish children dreamt of everyday misfortunes, both groups of Kurdish children dreamt of more life-threatening events.

The Kurdish children who experienced the most trauma had the most aggressive dreams of all three groups. Living in a dangerous environment as a child activates the threat-simulation system, said Revonsuo. He compared this to our immune system. If you are exposed to a lot of pathogens as a child, your immune system is in constant fighting mode and becomes trained for battle. If you live in a sterile environment, your immune system doesn't learn how to deal with viruses.

Face Your Fears

THREATS COME IN MANY forms, endangering us in different ways. There are the everyday threats that show up in our dreams, simulating various devastating scenarios. New mothers often imagine their newborns lost or hurt. For students, the threat could be failing an exam that could change the course of their lives.

Isabelle Arnulf and her team tested whether dreaming of an exam affected students' exam results. What if students dreamt of failing or acing an exam? How would this affect their marks? They gathered more than seven hundred students from Pierre and Marie Curie University in Paris who were preparing for the medical school entrance exam. Almost all students dreamt of the exam the night before and didn't sleep very well. About 78 percent of the exam dreams involved some sort of problem. Students dreamt of arriving late, not understanding the questions, or answering them incorrectly.

"I took the exam and made many mistakes," reported one participant. "Then, I had to explain to my parents that I failed and had to choose another orientation for my studies." Another student dreamt of having to take a plane to get to the exam. When the flight was cancelled, "I was obliged to go there in a camper on a sinuous mountain road during the night while watching the clock, which showed that the exam had started."[18] In their dreams, the students anticipated and prepared for possible problems on the day of the exam. All of their upset and distress paid off. Students who dreamt of the exam the night before as well as earlier in the term were more successful on the actual exam. Imagining potential pitfalls and testing out various solutions is akin to "how a chess player imagines all possible moves, particularly the moves leading to a loss, before selecting and playing the better move," explained the study's authors.[19] Just like the flight simulator, the learning in dreams comes from the variability and element of surprise.

As researchers discovered during the COVID-19 pandemic, it doesn't take long for the dreaming brain to test out a new threat. The pandemic "beautifully demonstrates how a new threat gets incorporated into our dream life quite quickly," said Revonsuo. Objects like face masks, which likely made rare appearances in dreams before March 2020, became fixtures in our dreams. Revonsuo dreamt of someone coughing in a crowded place. Realizing he didn't have his mask, Revonsuo searched for an escape route. This ability to recognize and prepare for different kinds of threats is what TST is all about. Whether it's contracting a virus, failing an exam, or a childhood nightmare of a thunderstorm, the dreaming brain tests a particular threat in many different ways, allowing the dreamer to practice alternative defenses.

I wondered what happens in the brain when we face our fears in our dreams. A few years ago, University of Geneva psychiatrist and researcher Lampros Perogamvros tested whether frightening dreams help us adapt to similar situations in our waking lives. Across two studies, they investigated two questions: Are the brain areas activated during frightening dreams the same regions activated when we experience fear in our waking lives? And if we experience a lot of fear in our dreams, does this affect how we react to fearful situations when we are awake?

To answer the first question, they looked at dream reports in NREM sleep (Stage 2) and REM sleep, identifying how often fear appeared in dreams. They found that frightening dreams in both NREM and REM sleep had heightened activity in the insula. REM sleep also had increased activation in the midcingulate cortex. These brain areas help us process upsetting or frightening events when we're awake. This showed that frightening experiences activate the same brain areas in dreams and in our waking lives.

For the second question, Perogamvros looked at the dream diaries of participants and asked them questions about their dreams. They found that more fear in dreams was associated with lower responses to fearful situations when they were awake. Using fMRI, they discovered that participants who experienced a lot of fear in their dreams had heightened activity in their medial prefrontal cortex when they were awake and faced fear-inducing stimuli. By facing fear in their dreams, they were better able to deal with fear in their waking lives. The findings supported the idea that dreams help with emotional regulation. In addition, they showed how frightening dreams help us prepare, or adapt, to risks in real life.[20]

I wanted to figure out where neutral or positive dreams fit into the Threat Simulation Theory. How could our non-threatening dreams be important for survival? Revonsuo told me how he had reflected on this idea for a long time. After the TST, he started looking at social bonding and social interactions within dreams. Decades of content analysis show that we are rarely alone in our dreams. Why is that? he wondered. Maybe the flip side of the negativity bias is a sociality bias, thought Revonsuo. This offered both sides of the equation that we required during evolutionary history. "We needed to survive the life-threatening and physically threatening dangers in our environment," he explained. "But we also needed to have skills in social bonding and social interaction."

In 2015, Revonsuo published his Social Simulation Theory (SST). He showed how in dreams, we create these social situations to practice interacting with others so we can develop much-needed relationships. Similar to a video game, our avatar stars in the virtual reality of our dreams. We meet other simulated characters whom we may love or fear, help or fight. "In our dreams, we live rich and colourful social lives," explained Revonsuo, "even if only simulated ones."[21] Similar to the TST, the SST focuses on practicing and preparing for what might await us during the day. Maybe it's testing out a difficult conversation with your boss or maybe you are navigating a new relationship. This rethinks the concept of survival.

Chapter Six

What Dreams Are
Made Of

SOME YEARS AGO ON A SNOWY MARCH EVENING, MY HUSBAND
and I found ourselves peering out the mud-streaked windows of a bus, looking for the Hôpital du Sacré-Cœur de Montréal. We were about a half-hour's
drive outside of downtown Montreal, riding through the suburbs north of
the city. The bus driver announced the stop for the hospital, and we stepped
onto a dark street. Perched on a hill, set far back from the road and the
flickering streetlight above us, was an old brick building. There wasn't the
usual bustle of hospital activity. No flurry of ambulances and attendants or
visitors milling about the front doors. It was just the two of us in front of the
hospital's towering iron gates.

On the roof above the main entrance was a statue of Mary with outstretched arms, her stance mirroring the heavy cross behind her. A spotlight illuminated her silhouette, clad in heavy robes, creating a stark
contrast against the black backdrop of the night. My gaze remained fixed
on Mary as we bumped our suitcase up the long driveway. Only the crunch
of stones and gravel beneath our winter boots interrupted the eerie stillness of the night.

We made our way along deserted halls, past an information booth that
was closed for the night, nodding to a security guard on our way by. It was
many years before a major renovation to modernize the facility, and the

hospital, built in 1927, felt like it was from another era. The surreal experience was much like a dream.

We took a small elevator to another empty hallway on a floor above and walked through the doors that read "silence SVP" (Quiet Please), into a modern wing with walls that displayed scientific papers. Behind closed doors were the offices of sleep researchers who had long gone home. One door remained unlocked, that of the Dream and Nightmare Laboratory where Dimitri and I would spend the night.

The lab consisted of a control area, bathroom, and two snug bedrooms, each furnished with a single bed, pine nightstand, and chair, all from Ikea. The bedrooms had some gadgets, too. A computer screen swung out from the wall across each bed like a vertical dinner tray, and an infrared camera and microphone, ready to record the next subject's night of sleep.

It was quite an unusual overnight getaway for the two of us. Dimitri had agreed to be the subject of a makeshift dream experiment so I could observe and investigate the memory sources of dreams. I've always wondered why we dream certain things at specific times in our lives. Does the sleeping brain pay more attention to certain types of memory? Does it prioritize events that have just happened and are still fresh in our minds? If that's the case, how do memories from our distant past find their way into our dreams? One often-cited study found that only 1 percent to 2 percent of reported dreams were exact replays of waking events with the same setting, characters, and plot. Yet more than half of the 299 dream reports included at least one element from waking experiences.[1] How, then, does the sleeping brain choose which fragments from waking life to explore in our dreams in new and unique ways?

Memory Trace

THERE ARE DIFFERENT KINDS of memory that help us navigate our interior and exterior worlds. Semantic memory encompasses facts and concepts. It's a combination of facts about the world and knowledge and beliefs about ourselves. My semantic memory tells me how to calculate t-tests and chi-square tests and reminds me that I found stats a really difficult course in grad school. Using my semantic memory, I can give my address to a cab driver without having to retrace the experience of learning the information.

Episodic memory helps us recall personal experiences including their times, places, and associated emotions. I use my episodic memory to recall my first snowboarding lesson outside of Banff, Alberta. I can picture how I tumbled backwards down the hill with my thick gloves flying in the air. Together, a semantic and an episodic memory make up a declarative memory, which is what we declare to be a truth. I remember that my wedding day was the hottest on record for that particular date in forty years. I know this because someone told me, even though I no longer remember who it was. Whether a declarative memory is actually true is another matter.

Procedural memory is a kind of implicit, long-term memory that helps us remember skills and perform tasks unconsciously. The constant drills in my high school typing course taught me the letter positions on my keyboard so that I can type this sentence without looking down. Yet if you asked me which letter sits above my left ring finger, I couldn't answer right away. I'd have to imagine typing a word like "why" to determine that it's the letter w. Procedural memory is what helps us climb on the bike that's been collecting dust in the garage and take off down the street as if we rode every day. It's a behind-the-scenes director waiting in the wings until she's needed.

Several studies associate the time of night with the recentness of a memory that we revisit in a dream. One study investigated the memory sources of dreams across all four stages of sleep. Twenty healthy subjects were awakened in NREM and REM sleep and asked to report their dreams. More than half of the dreams involved recent episodic memories, typically from the previous day, while 30 percent of dreams had distant memories. Just over 30 percent of dreams included semantic memories, those memories that involve facts and concepts. The researchers found that dreams during Stage 1 and REM incorporated more memory sources, which might be attributed to the creative brainstorming of Stage 1 and the abstract combinations of memories in REM sleep.

When they looked at memory sources in relation to the time of night, the researchers found that recent memories appeared earlier while more remote memories showed up later in the night. Recent memories decreased after the first third of the night and this change wasn't affected by the stage of sleep. So as we move deeper into the night and farther away from the previous day, the memories that play out in our dreams become more distant. One possibility is that NREM and REM sleep work together as well as in sequence to help process memories, which become more remote across a night's sleep.[2] It can be difficult, though, to place certain memories. Someone might dream of a car crash and relate it to a movie they watched recently. Or maybe the dream sparks the memory of a car accident that happened years earlier.

A Night at the Sleep Lab

THE DREAM AND NIGHTMARE Laboratory is one of the world's leading dream research facilities dedicated to investigating and advancing dream science. The lab's director, Tore Nielsen, and his team have done numerous studies on memory and dreams. Nielsen is a professor in the department of psychiatry and addictology at the Université de Montréal. Over several decades, he has studied many aspects of dreaming, including the dreams of sleep onset. These first few minutes of the sleep cycle are characterized by strong, crisp images rather than meandering plots. The Japanese psychologist and sleep researcher Tadao Hori identified unique EEG patterns of brain waves during sleep onset and defined nine stages within the first period of sleep.

Across several studies, Nielsen has focused on Substages 4 and 5 of sleep onset, when the childlike scribbles of alpha waves—the brain waves connected to relaxed and meditative states—flatten out to a bumpy line with the occasional hiccup, and the brain teeters on the edge of waking and sleep. This is when dreams begin to take shape. In one study, most sleep onset dream reports fell into either Substage 4 or 5. At this point, subjects were awakened and asked what they were thinking about. What images flashed behind their closed lids? The researchers investigated why certain memories are chosen during sleep onset.

During our sleepover at the lab, Dimitri followed a similar protocol to subjects in a study on memory and dreams. This included performing a virtual reality exercise, watching an animated film clip, and keeping a dream diary for ten days. Before bed, Dimitri changed into his pajamas and relaxed while electrodes were pasted onto certain points of his skull to measure brain wave activity. This included two along the occipital lobes at the back of his head that would measure alpha activity when he first lay down for the night. When the jumpy brain waves flattened out, it would signal that Dimitri had drifted off to sleep. Electrodes were placed on his chin to measure muscle atonia, or cessation of movement, which is associated with REM sleep. Two electrodes were placed on his temples to gauge his facial expressions during sleep. I learned that people often frown when they have nightmares. An electrode on the front of his chest would measure his heart rate and rhythm. Another electrode attached to his leg would report any restless leg movements. An electrode on his arm would also measure his movement and alert us if he awoke.

Once the set-up was complete, the electrodes were fed into a small green box at his hip, which let Dimitri wander around until bedtime. When it was lights out, the box would be plugged into a wire in his bedroom to send electrical signals to the computer in the control area. These signals transform into skittish, squiggly, and rolling lines, creating a digital sleep pattern of body and brain wave activity.

The lab door swung open, and Philippe Stenstrom, then a PhD candidate in psychology, walked in, dressed in jeans, a bulky sweater, and mountain boots. Stenstrom was our technician for the night and would monitor Dimitri's sleep study. He hadn't had a chance to eat, and dove into a box of Chips Ahoy cookies. When I asked what he was studying, he talked about his fascination with memory and sleep, specifically episodic memory, that kind of reminiscence for the time, place, and emotionality of past events. He described episodic memory as the essence of dreaming. He explained how dreaming is almost like another form of episodic recollection. When awake, we transport ourselves back to memorable past events. During dreams, we might use the same processes to achieve memory recall. In the lab, Stenstrom was working with Nielsen to study the memory sources of dreams.

Exhausted and groggy, Dimitri retreated to his bedroom. Propped up against the headboard with a Medusa-like headful of wires, Dimitri pulled the computer screen from the wall toward him. At this point, his brain waves weren't being recorded. Stenstrom set up an animated video clip to test Dimitri's waking memory. We would then see if Dimitri dreamt about the short video later on or during subsequent nights. I sat in the control room and watched the same clip on another computer.

Film Noir

IT WAS NIGHTTIME, AND we watched the snow fall. The camera panned across the boxy skyscraper silhouette of a city suggestive of New York. The scene flipped to a man in a fedora. He sat in a dark office in front of a large window through which falling snowflakes cast their shadows. A white cat sat on a radiator, and a close-up of a magnifying glass scanned a document. The office setting changed to an aerial map of the city. In the montage of images, a man ran down a flight of stairs. Once he reached the street, the man looked up at a fire escape where another cat, grey this time, was perched, holding the hat between its teeth. The cat released the hat, which the man caught before he ran away. Cut to the man in a train station where he raced along a platform to catch a moving train. At the last second, the man jumped, grabbing onto the side of the train. Aboard, he knocked on a compartment. When he burst through the door, the man came face-to-face with a woman pointing a gun at him. For several seconds, we remained frozen in this moment. Then our screens went blank.

Stenstrom asked Dimitri to type out whatever he could remember of the last sixty seconds of the clip. By asking him to focus on the conclusion, Stenstrom had Dimitri reconstruct the film in the same way that people recall their dreams. When we wake up in the morning, we don't usually remember our dream in chronological order. We think of the last image that flashed through our minds, and then we work backwards, trying to remember what came before.

Dimitri sat up in bed without typing, at a loss for words. The film had felt so fast and jumbled that it was difficult to remember the last image or even most of the clip. After a few moments, he typed, "The man is on a train and enters a compartment and is grabbed or hit or attacked by someone who is hiding in the compartment. The person appears to be a woman and may be dressed in some sort of superhero outfit. The man is dressed in a 1940s-style suit and fedora hat. Everything is black and white." Dimitri filled in some other details. "There are snowflakes falling in a city landscape, much like a comic-book setting—maybe Gotham," he wrote. "There is a man sitting in a chair in the dark in an office. We are looking at him from above." Dimitri remembered the magnifying glass that scanned a document, and the train that moved from the foreground into the dark background.

Stenstrom asked Dimitri to watch the film clip a second time to see if he could improve his recall. At the end of the viewing, Dimitri was once again left with the image of a woman pointing a gun at a man before the shot faded to black. This time, Dimitri could remember farther back into the scene. "The man runs down the stairs of the train station (he has a gun in his hand) and reaches the platform just as the train is departing the station. He runs and jumps with great difficulty (almost falling) and grabs onto the back of the train. Cut to the man standing in front of a compartment door." He felt confident that the scene continued as he first remembered it.

As Dimitri pondered the rest of the clip, he recalled the white cat perched on the radiator and the grey cat that dropped the fedora from the fire escape to the man below. Dimitri focused on the mood of the clip. "These scenes are all dark and cold-feeling," he typed. "The movie has a film noir feel to it with all of the attending feelings of high drama and stylized atmosphere. Style over substance."

The purpose of this kind of exercise is to improve dream reports of subjects. The retelling of a dream, like a dream itself, is a very subjective process. A dream is worth ten thousand words easily, Nielsen told me, but which ten thousand words will subjects choose to describe it? A visual person might zoom in on the look of a dream while an auditory person might focus on the sounds that accompany images. When asked to recount dreams, people go into tell-a-good-story mode, said Nielsen, who looks for details on how people navigate their dream worlds. How do they turn their heads or reach for an object? Do they walk through or around doors?

In one study, Nielsen and his team taught participants to focus on our non-obvious daytime actions that use our perception. They had participants report perceptual details from the film clip and then asked subjects to report them for their dreams. After the training, subjects reported more perception-like details. The idea was to try and expose part of the infrastructure of dreaming that usually goes unnoticed in typical dream reports, Nielsen explained. Reflecting on these details allowed the researchers to compare people's actions in waking and dreaming states.

Dreams are a kind of virtual reality that allows us to experience things similar to waking life. In dreams, our world is structured differently. But we are using similar perceptual tools that we use when we are awake, explained Nielsen. "The object of perception is our own memory terrain," he said. "We're looking around in a different vault." Instead of replaying entire episodic memories, we incorporate details from waking life into our dreams. We reconstruct things, putting bits and pieces of memories together in new ways. Nielsen compared the process of dreaming to improv when an actor or musician reacts in the moment. Dreamers also act on the spot, he told me. Information is thrown at them and they put it together in new scenarios. But unlike comic improv, dreams aren't usually funny. Often, they're negative or frightening.

With negative dreams, we evoke fragments or feelings of fear-based memories. One idea is that dreaming is designed to extinguish fear memories. In dreams, we revisit frightening scenarios while our dreaming brains are working in a different state, which changes how we think, feel, and react to fearful situations. To extinguish a fear, we don't simply forget it. Instead, we create a new memory trace, or safety memory, that competes with and eventually overrides the old memory, Nielsen told me. The previous memory remains filed away somewhere and can be reactivated in certain circumstances.

We talked about the example of Pavlov's dogs, which learned to associate the ringing of a bell with food. The dogs became so conditioned that they salivated when they heard the bell, even when there was no food in sight. An unusual thing happened in 1924, when the dogs' kennel was flooded. The dogs were trapped for many days, trying to keep their heads above water. When they were finally rescued, the frightened animals became depressed. They had no interest in food and stopped salivating at the ring of a bell. Over time, their conditioning returned but would once again vanish when water trickled into the room. The dogs' fear had overpowered their conditioned learning.

So how do you create a new memory to override a fear? Imagine that you are doing the dishes and you slice your hand with a sharp knife. When you see a sharp knife after that, fear surges within you. You can't forget what happened, just like when I tried to slice a frozen bagel and ended up cutting my palm. "Emotion enhances learning," Nielsen explained. "The glue of episodic memories is probably emotion." Suddenly, you are hesitant or even afraid to wash the dishes. The sink might even become something associated with your fear. The way to extinguish the fear is to create new memories of knives in different and safe contexts. Maybe you imagine cutting bread away from the sink or using different kinds of knives, say a butter knife, and you do this without cutting yourself. Over time, you neutralize the fear associated with the object by creating new memories around it.

In a way, this is what dreams do. They put together the most incongruous things. Imagine a dream in which someone approaches you in a dark alley. Then suddenly, there's an ice cream truck and someone hands you a chocolate-dipped cone. You fill in the details of the person's face and realize it's a friend. That initial fear is recast in your mind, being associated with ice cream and a good friend. It doesn't seem so scary after all. The process breaks down when someone suffers from a traumatic experience, which, in the case of PTSD, is often revisited in dreams without any resolution or relief.

The Edge of Sleep

FOR MY VISIT TO the lab, we focused on retracing memories during sleep onset, when Dimitri first drifted off. The plan was for Stenstrom to waken Dimitri four times during sleep onset to see what was on his mind and try to connect the hypnagogic images with memories. The images of sleep onset are dreamlike in that they are visual and auditory. But they don't have the complex plots of dreams later in the night.

As Dimitri settled in a few minutes before midnight—my barrage of questions had kept the subject up later than usual—I sat down beside Stenstrom. The infrared camera showed Dimitri moving around, trying to find a comfortable position. He hadn't slept well the night before, and he was exhausted from the six-hour trip by train, subway, and bus that had brought us from Toronto that morning. He drifted off within minutes.

Stenstrom pointed to Dimitri's alpha waves, which had unraveled from tight scribbles to hiccupy ripples. This kind of languid brain wave is associated with the hypnagogic imagery of sleep onset. "Whether he's sleeping or not is unclear," he said. "It's cool. It's at the threshold of sleep." His brain waves flattened out even more. Stenstrom explained that we were looking for five seconds of this activity. "He's getting close now. He's very tired," said Stenstrom. After several seconds of the low-tide waves, Stenstrom pushed a button on his computer. The microphone in Dimitri's room emitted a tinny beeping sound, waking him from his short-lived slumber.

"What was on your mind?" asked Stenstrom in a deep, soothing voice fit for a sleep lab. It took a few seconds for Dimitri to orient himself. "Hitler," he answered. "I was picturing Hitler with his signature moustache. Then Hitler changed into my uncle Jos, who has a moustache that curls up at the edges. Then there were flamingoes. And then I had some vague thoughts about work."

Stenstrom asked if he could connect these images to anything that had happened lately. Before falling asleep, Dimitri was reading a book on the Second World War and earlier in the day, we'd been talking about his uncle. So he connected the two by their moustaches. At first, he couldn't imagine where the flamingoes had come from, but then he remembered our recent chat about staying home over winter break instead of visiting my parents in Maui. This reminded him of our morning running route past a hotel with a group of resident flamingoes that ignored the passing crowd. The fleeting thoughts of work might have stemmed from a going-away party he had attended the previous night.

Dimitri was left to fall back asleep, which he did within minutes. At 12:16 a.m., Stenstrom identified the brain waves of sleep onset and buzzed Dimitri out of his slumber. This time, Dimitri told us about a beautiful woman in a puffy white gown, heavy with lace. Inside the dress was a cat, which turned into a dog, then a man, then a woman again with bright red lipstick and a tower of bleach blond curls pulled high above her powdered face. The image transformed into two jagged rows of lines that chomped down like teeth. He described the same dark feeling he had when he'd watched the film clip. When asked about possible connections to the extravagantly dressed woman, Dimitri recalled a subway poster of a woman with porcelain skin and stained red lips wearing an outlandish white dress. About a week earlier, we had watched Sofia Coppola's *Marie Antoinette*, but Dimitri didn't mention this.

Just before 1 a.m., Dimitri burrowed under the covers and tried to steal a few more minutes of sleep. Stenstrom noticed that Dimitri was having a period of REM-like sleep, which doesn't typically happen during sleep onset. His eyes darted back and forth, yet his chin wasn't paralyzed as it would be during REM sleep. This might mean that he was having more vivid imagery than usual during the first stage of sleep. Awakened, Dimitri described big creatures with long necks and wide gaping mouths that reminded him of the Loch Ness monster. They changed into Venus flytraps, then into creeping spiders. Then he saw a pug and wondered if it was my cousin's dog, Tulip. He remembered bumping into my cousin Rob a few days earlier.

Left alone again, Dimitri fell asleep quickly. Then at 1:10 a.m., Dimitri was awakened for the last time. He described peering inside a luxurious leather briefcase, but nothing was there. Then he saw a group of faceless coworkers talking about him, wondering if he was going to take "the documents." He looked down and saw that he held some rolled-up papers. Then he imagined going to a friend's office to hide them. When asked to reflect on his dream, Dimitri didn't hesitate. He had decided to take a new job and was preoccupied by how the news would be taken.

Dream Life

THE NEXT MORNING, NIELSEN walked into the lab, his blue eyes greeting us through rectangular glasses. Cradling a travel mug of coffee, he looked as groggy as us, having been hard at work on a grant proposal that was due the next day. We sat down and worked on connecting Dimitri's dreams with what was happening in his waking life. We talked about Hitler appearing along with his uncle Jos. Sure, Dimitri had been reading a book on the war before falling asleep. Yet after a few minutes of brainstorming, he connected more deep-rooted memories. Dimitri grew up listening to his father's stories of life in Holland during the war. His uncle Jos was born during that time. The week before, Dimitri and I had talked about how his dad would enjoy living in Holland again after his retirement, speaking his native language and immersing himself in Dutch culture.

Scenes from the film clip hadn't played out in his dreams, as expected. Our dreaming brain doesn't simply hit replay on memories. Yet there was the random appearance of a cat, and the same dark feeling that Dimitri experienced when he watched the clip. The memory traces were from different days in the previous week. This showed that Dimitri wasn't simply drawing on a single episodic memory.

Nielsen told me about the Dream Lag Effect, a finding about one mechanism that influences how—or when—dreams incorporate memories. There is a good chance that experiences we have during the day will in some way show up in our dreams that night. It's what Freud called day residue. The next night, our chances of dreaming about the previous day's experiences drop significantly. During nights three, four, and five, we probably won't dream of those experiences. Yet on nights six, seven, and eight, there is a good chance that we will revisit them. This is when we get the dream lag effect.

Why does this happen? It might relate to the workings of the hippocampus, which helps transfer experiences from short-term to long-term memory. It takes time to give a memory permanence. It's thought to take about a week for the memory transfer, and this parallels what Nielsen has found in the lag effect of some dreams. It's a bit of a mystery as to why some memories go underground during nights three, four, and five. But Nielsen believes that the memories the brain chooses to revisit later are characterized by their spatial, social, and emotional qualities. We tend to revisit powerful memories that, for many possible reasons, leave a lasting impression.[3]

Nielsen used an interactive maze-like video game to study the spatial and social characteristics of lagged memories. Two groups of subjects participated: one group played the game on a high-definition television (HDTV) and the other group played the same game using a virtual-reality headset. The images seen on the headset's built-in screen appeared grainier than those on the HDTV while the images on the TV had a wider panorama. Both groups played the game for hours, and their dreams were studied for the following ten days.

Nielsen discovered that the dream lag occurred for all of the subjects as they'd been actively involved in the experience, using a mouse or headset to navigate their movements. Those who had cyber sickness and became nauseous had a stronger lag effect, dreaming vividly of the experience. Just over a week after the exercise in the lab, they dreamt of the interactive maze. The TV group had a lag effect of one more day than the virtual-reality group. The TV condition was more engaging, causing the participants to dream about it more during the nights immediately following the exposure, and then about a week after that as well, he said. The day residue and dream-lag curve were shifted a couple of days because of this, explained Nielsen.

The day after our sleepover in the lab, Dimitri participated in a similar virtual-reality exercise. His mission was to find his way out of a complex underground labyrinth. He slipped on a headset and began to move by using a joystick. From the control room, I watched him shift his body and turn his head as he manipulated his player through the maze. The passageways looked maddeningly indistinguishable, and as he travelled in circles, he searched for landmarks to get his bearings.

The maze opened onto a junkyard where he balanced himself across a tightrope of old, decaying boards of wood. Suddenly, he was face-to-face with another player who had been skewered by a large spike. "I feel horrible," said Dimitri, when asked what the experience was like. "I want to get out of here as soon as possible." For several minutes, he traveled underground through crumbling passageways that eventually opened onto a mountainous, snowy area and then returned him underground to a maze of bridges suspended above bubbling hot lava. After nineteen tiring minutes, he jumped into the lava, ending the game.

On our long train ride home, I wondered what next week's dreams would hold. Would Dimitri imagine himself back in the virtual labyrinth, turning from the sight of the man stabbed with a steel spike? Or would he incorporate images from the dark, moody film clip?

Every morning for the next ten days, I woke him up, excited to hear about his dreams. Nothing from our night in the lab resurfaced. Until day eight, when our shrill alarm interrupted his strange dream. Dimitri sat up in bed and described being wheeled into a hospital on a gurney. He had come down with a very serious condition: he couldn't remember any of his dreams. His sleeping mind was blank.

Memories don't come to us as exact replays of events. They aren't like a video camera with an on/off switch, explained Nielsen. "We can enter and exit a memory where we like, remembering different things during one recollection and other things during another," he said. In dreams, memory elements are included in a similar, fragmented way, he explained. Nielsen pointed out that less than 2 percent of dreams replay episodic memories in their entirety, and even those don't likely include all of a memory's elements. Dreams are creative reconstructions of our memories.

Next on my exploration of dreams and memory, I looked at how sleep and dreams might strengthen and integrate memories into our vast catalogue of remembered thoughts and experiences. To do this, I found myself speeding down a snow-covered mountain, even though I hadn't clipped on ski boots for years.

Chapter Seven

Making Memories Stick

SOME YEARS AGO, I FOUND MYSELF STANDING ATOP A SNOW-covered mountain, surrounded by a vast cerulean sky and craggy alpine peaks. I clicked my heavy ski boots into their bindings, slipped on my goggles, and inched toward the mountain's edge. My gaze followed the tips of my skis down the steep run as I tried to quell my vertigo. It was a long way down. But I wasn't worried about breaking a leg, even though I hadn't downhill skied in years. Any wipeouts would be painless because none of this was really happening. I was actually at the Beth Israel Deaconess Medical Center in Boston, playing a video game.

I was there to investigate why certain experiences, like an immersive video game, become memories that we choose to dream about. In the last chapter, we saw how recent episodic memories reappear during the first few minutes of sleep. Now we're adding implicit memory to the mix. Implicit memory lets us recall things unconsciously and includes procedural memory, which helps us perform tasks instinctively, like riding a bike or braving the slopes. I hadn't downhill skied in years and I'd never played a skiing arcade game. So this experience would involve procedural learning and dust off some old implicit memories.

The makeshift arcade was care of Robert Stickgold, a professor at Harvard Medical School and founder of Harvard's Center Centre for Sleep and Cognition. He is an expert on memory and dreams and has been studying sleep and dreams for decades, including how dreams help process important and emotional experiences. I had the chance to test this when I visited Stickgold and spent many hours in a converted storage closet playing Alpine Racer II, which catapults players down mountainous hills at breakneck speed.

At the time of my visit, I was six months pregnant, and my balance was more off than usual. I stepped onto the machine and planted my feet firmly in the foot pedals that would angle my movement down the hill. My fingers encircled black rubber hand grips that felt like the ones on my ski poles. A large screen displayed the back of my player, suited in a puffy parka, cap, and gloves. Ready to kick up some snow, I pressed the red start button. "3-2-1 GO!" shouted the announcer, and I took off. I pivoted the foot pedals, trying to keep on course. Within moments I crashed into a mountain. "Watch out!" screamed the announcer. Dusting myself off, I launched myself down the hill into a series of jumps. Somehow, I stayed upright after a triple jump that made my stomach somersault like the sheer drop of a roller coaster. I ducked under a bridge, crouching on the pedals. Veering away from a tree, I tightened my grasp on the hand grips.

I fixed my gaze on the screen, forgetting the buzz of activity around me. I shifted my body, transferring my weight as if I were really skiing. My next meetings were pushed out of my mind. I was inside the game, and nothing else could compete for my attention. After an hour of virtual skiing, my speed began to improve as I anticipated the course. Ready for the hairpin turns, I finally made it down the hill without wiping out. I spent a long time trying to beat my score. When I finally stepped off the machine, I felt woozy, as if I were still in the game. I steadied myself against a pile of boxes and regained my balance, planting myself firmly back on earth.

I spent the rest of the day immersed in research for this book, and I forgot about my stint as an alpine racer. Exhausted, I went back to my hotel with some lukewarm takeout. When I turned out the light that night, I wondered if I was going to dream about playing the game, which made me convinced that wanting to do just that would prevent it. There was so much new information to process from the day, not to mention the stack of scientific studies that I was working my way through.

As I began to drift off, I dipped in between this world and sleep. My mind shuffled through images from the day. I lost touch with my tired body, tucked under crisp hotel sheets. Suddenly, there was that somersault in my stomach again as if I were falling from a great height. I was back on the ski hill, maneuvering through a maze of trees. I wiped out, spraying a wave of powdery snow. I wasn't *playing* the game, operating the foot pedals and hand grips. I didn't see the large screen or the red button that I had pressed continuously to have another try. I was inside the game, *living* it. I kept repeating the moments that didn't go so well. The tricky jumps and turns that had sent me rolling headfirst down the hill. But what about those runs where I had managed to stay on my feet?

I woke up with lots of questions for Stickgold. That blustery winter morning in Boston, I found Stickgold hunched over his computer, sorting through the day's overwhelming mass of emails. He swiveled his chair toward the door to greet me. He had rolled up the sleeves of his brown-and-olive checkered shirt, glasses dangled from a string around his neck, and his cellphone case, attached to his jeans, read "Bob." A Rubik's Cube and other games designed to tax the brain lined the windowsill. Stuck to his filing cabinet was a magnet that read "consciousness, that confusing time between naps" and another that said "Can't sleep. Clowns will eat me."

I sat down across from Stickgold to ask about the previous night's dreams. It was remarkable how he was able to predict the kind of images that had flooded my mind as I fell asleep. They were the moments when I was really involved in the game, when I was emotionally invested in how I was doing. Stickgold explained that we often dream about what happened during the day that was important and unsettled. So that's why I kept reliving those hairpin turns that sent me tumbling down the hill. Why do some memories seem more important to us than others? How does the brain choose which thoughts and experiences to dream about? To figure this out, I first had to understand how a memory is formed, stored, and recalled.

How to Make a Memory

A MEMORY ISN'T STORED in one specific location in the brain. Imagine information housed in many areas that come together to create a cohesive story. Memory is an intangible process by which we trigger networks within the brain to reconstruct things that have happened—or we imagine to have happened—days, months, or years earlier. We hold onto impressions of the past. Since memory is by nature subjective, our memories are actually reconstructions of past events. Just ask a couple to recall details about their honeymoon. Each will likely insist that their version of events is accurate, even if it's wildly different than their partner's. This is partly because we focus on differing aspects and can have vastly different interpretations of the same experience. It also doesn't help that our memory can deceive us, especially over time.

I have this vivid memory of being four years old and intent on helping my mother with the ironing. I picture myself in our kitchen, staring up at the iron, which was heating up on the ironing board. Standing on the balls of my feet, I reached for the iron and pulled it toward me. Then I plunked down onto the kitchen floor and began to iron the skin on the underside of my forearm. My mom came into the room, scooped me up, and drove to the emergency room where my dad was working. When I brought up the story recently with my mom, I discovered that I never went to the hospital. The moment she noticed the raw, red outline of an iron on my skin, my father had walked through the door after his hospital shift, and he tended to my arm in our bathroom. One material truth remains: the accident left no scar.

The day after the American space shuttle *Challenger* exploded in 1986, a group of psychology students was asked to record how they'd learned of the event and where they were when it happened. Three years later, they were asked the same questions as well as an additional one: How confident were they in their memories? While all of the students gave themselves either perfect or near-perfect scores for recall, one-third of them were in fact wrong in their reconstructions. The answers given three years later didn't match their responses from 1986.[1]

Misleading witness accounts can have costly consequences. An example is the witness statements from the 1995 Oklahoma bombing, a deadly act of domestic terrorism masterminded by Timothy McVeigh, who was eventually executed for the mass murder. McVeigh used a truck bomb to carry out the crime. Workers from Elliott's Body Shop, where he rented the vehicle, were called in as witnesses in the case. Of the three employees who identified McVeigh renting the truck, only one person said initially that he was accompanied by another man. Later on, the other two witnesses changed their stories to describe a second man. This set off a police search for a man authorities now believe to be nonexistent. Months later, the witness who first recalled an accomplice retracted his statement, saying he might have been thinking of a different customer who had nothing to do with the incident.[2] So what really happened? McVeigh visited the body shop alone.

This kind of "memory conformity" can happen when a self-assured witness sways others, creating a collaborative account of events. Of course, shared details can be accurate as well as misleading. In one study, Fiona Gabbert recruited sixty students and sixty older adults. Subjects saw one of two film clips of a girl dropping off a borrowed book, shown from different angles to reflect differing perspectives of witnesses. Half of the older and younger subjects watched alone while the other half were each paired with another witness. Those in the co-witness group thought they were watching the same clip, but a barrier prevented them from realizing they saw the situation from different angles. After the video, subjects filled out a questionnaire, with half working on it alone and the other half working with their co-witness. Certain questions could only be answered correctly by those who saw the clip from the first perspective. For example, they were asked to identify the title of the girl's book, which was visible only in one of the videos.

Gabbert found that both the student and older adult co-witnesses incorporated information from fellow participants. In fact, 71 percent of witnesses who discussed the event included information from their conversation. A shocking 60 percent of subjects in the co-witness group decided the girl was guilty of a crime that they didn't witness. Interestingly, age was not a factor for memory conformity. This shows how people's versions of events can change when they're given additional information. It demonstrates that memory is a self-constructed illusion built from selected material that is stuck together with interpretive glue.

How do memories, fictious and real, form in the brain? The hippocampus, the horseshoe-shaped structure in the temporal lobe, helps to organize and retrieve memories and is integral in making memories long-term. It knows where to find the different components of memories, including spatial and auditory information. Neuroscientist György Buzsáki compared the hippocampus to a librarian in his book *Rhythms of the Brain*. Imagine the cortex is a massive library and the hippocampus is its very own librarian, he explained. The hippocampus finds components of memories, puts them together, and pulls them off our library shelves so we can remember. The amygdala, the almond-shaped structure that is also in the temporal lobe, is integral to our emotional responses like anger and fear. It helps create emotional memories. This makes me think of how the emotions woven into a memory often determine whether I'll remember it.

I'll never forget the surge of fear when our car hit a patch of black ice one Christmas Eve and skated off a two-lane country road, narrowly missing a guardrail. Luckily, the panic and fear surrounding this memory have dampened over time. I'm able to remember that day without experiencing the same intense emotions, as Matthew Walker and Els van der Helm point out is common, in their model of dreams as overnight therapy. They showed that when we dream during REM sleep, we sleep to remember the details of an experience while we sleep to forget, or ease, its emotional sting.[3]

Many studies point to the connection between sleep and memory consolidation, specifically how sleep helps to strengthen, store, and integrate memories. It's thought that while we sleep, the hippocampus and neocortex work together to strengthen new memories and integrate them with recollections of the past.

Memory is a complex process that involves learning, or encoding, information, then storing this information and later retrieving it. New information is placed in our working memory, which is a type of short-term memory that holds data temporarily. Imagine my car breaks down and I need roadside assistance. I Google the number and repeat it to myself a few times so I can tap it into my phone. If I get distracted by an incoming text while I'm repeating the number, I'll probably have to start the process again.

The Memory Collector

IF I WANT TO remember something over time, I'll need to store it within my long-term memory. Imagine that I'm at a party and I'm introduced to Mrs. Smith. I shake her hand, my brain producing a pattern of neural activity as I register her name. As we talk, another pattern of activity takes in her features: the sharp outline of her face, her gold-flecked hazel eyes, and her auburn corkscrew curls. A different area of my brain creates my emotional reaction to her. Maybe I feel anxious talking to a good friend of my boss: an emotional reaction that has its own pattern of activity. All of these visual, auditory, sensory, and emotional bits of information are housed in different areas of the brain. The hippocampus works with the neocortex to strengthen the connections between pieces of information to create a memory. When we first learn new information, the hippocampus helps us process and retain recent memories. As time progresses, the neocortex binds pieces of information together, shedding its dependence on the hippocampus.

The neurons creating patterns for Mrs. Smith's face and name work together to create one complete picture. These patterns of brain activity are being performed by neural hardware that has its connections set from past experiences. Over time, we learn how to remember. When I meet Mrs. Smith and learn her name, processing the emotion of this new encounter, changes in neural activity occur, which then result in the formation of a new memory. I've met other people with hazel eyes and curly hair, but when my brain combines these aspects with a feeling of nervousness as well as other thoughts and emotions from the cocktail party, a new memory trace is laid down.

How do we make a memory stick? To give permanence to a memory, we need to encode it more deeply. We can do this by associating it with other memories. My son's phone number was easy to memorize because it has a similar pattern to my own. When learning something new, we search our library of past experiences and knowledge to see where it fits into what we already know. This is partly why two people—like the couple recalling their honeymoon—can have such conflicting memories of the same event.

If we encode new information, how do we forget what we learned? Let's say that a few months after the party, I run into Mrs. Smith on the street. I may have trouble remembering how I know her, let alone her name, when I see her out of context. I know we've met, because I recognize her face. Suddenly, I remember her name, and I blurt it out before my cheeks flush with embarrassment. As my mind compiles different patterns of activity, I piece together the night we met.

Or maybe she looks familiar, but I'm tongue-tied on her name. Perhaps I remember that it starts with an "S" and flip through the catalogue of names stored within my memory until I figure out it's Smith. If I can't recall her name, maybe it's because we didn't talk that long, or maybe I didn't think about her after that night, so I didn't strengthen the connections to create a lasting memory trace. As time passed, the neural connections creating the image of the party weakened. I'm left with a vague impression of her, like a rough sketch of how she looks, and, if I'm lucky, her name. Since we met, my brain has been busy learning and integrating new information with old thoughts and experiences. We don't replay memories like packaged scenes from a movie, complete with setting, dialogue, and plot. Sometimes we recognize the characters and essence of a story while forgetting names and details.

So how does the brain decide what to keep and what to discard? Stickgold thinks the brain looks for emotional salience, repetition, and recentness to decide whether to hold on to a memory. Take the dates that I gave birth to my kids. There are so many reasons why these days are meaningful to me, which strengthens the neural network of these particular memories. The same is true, though mundanely, for my banking PIN, which I tap into the machine every time I withdraw money. By contrast, I probably only remembered for a day or two which terminal I flew into on my trip to Boston to visit Stickgold. The information left my mind when it was no longer needed, having lost its recentness and its relevance. Then there are memories we can't seem to shake, no matter how hard we try. Memories infused with emotion, be it fear, joy, or embarrassment, leave their mark. As William James noted in 1890, "an impression may be so exciting emotionally as almost to leave a *scar* upon the cerebral tissues."[4]

How does sleep fit into the process? Which memories get front-of-the-line priority in our dreams? During sleep onset, the brain tags certain memories to revisit later in sleep. "Your brain is intentionally lining up things to work on later in the night," Stickgold told me. How does the brain decide what to tag during those first few minutes of sleep? There are several factors at play. Stickgold pointed to thoughts that are emotional or unsettled. As we fall asleep, our thoughts are often about "incomplete processes," he said. This could be a situation or conversation that didn't come to a neat and tidy conclusion. It could be as simple as replaying a recent conversation with your boss who'd said "good luck" on your presentation. "You might find yourself lying in bed trying to replay the precise nuance of his voice," said Stickgold.

While learning new knowledge or tasks could be flagged to work through during sleep, Stickgold doesn't think it's that simple. It might also have to do with emotional effect. We probably wouldn't dream of sitting in front of our computer for hours, memorizing word pairs. But if we kept crashing on this one turn in a virtual skiing game, there's a good chance it would show up in those brief, hypnagogic dreams at the start of the night.

Dream researchers have discovered the power of intentional, focused thinking. We can guide our thoughts as we fall asleep toward something as emotionally neutral as a tree. We now know that sleep onset isn't just about tagging memories. There is something magical that happens on the border between the waking and dreaming worlds, which I will investigate later in the book.

Jumping the Queue

A FAMILY TRIP TO Vermont inspired some of Stickgold's early experiments in sleep and memory. Several decades ago, Stickgold and his family hiked some trails along Camel's Hump, a four-thousand-foot mountain aptly named for its two-peaked profile. There was one area that required some climbing. One after another, they grasped the jagged rock, pulling themselves up the mountainside. That night, as Stickgold began to fall asleep, he found himself back on the mountain, grabbing onto rock just as he had done earlier that day. He wasn't thinking about the hours they had spent walking along the path. He was reliving the difficult passage on the trail and felt the sensation of rock underneath his hands. He awoke, thinking about the experience, then fell back asleep. As he drifted off, it happened again. He tried to focus on a manuscript he was writing, but the sensation of his hands gripping rock pushed the paper out of his mind. He awoke later in the night, and as he drifted off again, he tried to get the climb to reappear. Yet the sensation had slipped from his hands. What was it about the timing of the recollection? Why was Stickgold able to conjure the images when he first fell asleep?

A few days later, Stickgold rafted with his family down a river in Vermont. That night, he relived the feeling of crashing over the rapids. The following year, he took his son downhill skiing. After a day on the slopes, Stickgold drifted off to sleep. He found himself back on the ski hill, edging his way down the tricky run. He told his son, who had been dreaming of the day as well, suspended on the ski lift with his skis dangling mid-air.

Stickgold wondered how he could study the impact of such an engrossing experience as climbing a mountain or braving rapids in a safe, controlled environment. During a lab discussion, one of Stickgold's students described vivid images after playing Tetris, a video game that has players fit colourful blocks together as they fall down the screen. One Christmas, Stickgold had played a game similar to Tetris in which players assemble a jumble of cascading bricks. That Christmas night, Stickgold had drifted off while he imagined bricks falling. Stickgold found other Tetris players who'd had similar nighttime experiences. The safe, engaging game proved to be an ideal experience to study.

In 2000, Stickgold and his team gathered twenty-seven subjects, dividing them into three groups. The novice group had never played Tetris. The expert group had played between fifty and five hundred hours of Tetris before the experiment. The third group of subjects had amnesia and were thought to be new to Tetris. With damage to their hippocampus, they couldn't remember recent experiences. In some instances, though, people with amnesia can retrieve recent information, much to their own surprise.

When I asked Stickgold if this was really possible, he pointed to the work of Édouard Claparède. In the 1800s, the Swiss physician conducted memory studies of patients with amnesia. One of Claparède's patients retained some past memories, but it seemed like she couldn't form new ones. The woman couldn't remember meeting Claparède when he entered the room repeatedly. Then the physician decided to mix up their usual meet-and-greet. He hid a pin between two fingers, which pricked her skin when they shook hands. The next time Claparède greeted her with an outstretched hand, she refused to shake it. Asked why, she answered that sometimes pins are hidden in people's hands. The memory was stored somewhere within her brain.[5]

It's possible that people without a properly functioning hippocampus can tap into implicit memories to perform procedural tasks. For example, someone with amnesia can practice typing every day and have no recollection. They might even believe that they can't type. But if you ask them to type their name, their fingers might fly across the keys, much to their surprise, as they type out their name without a glance at the keyboard.

Now let's see what happened with the subjects who played many hours of Tetris, including those with amnesia. Over several nights in the lab, subjects reported what was on their mind at different points in the night. Nine of the twelve new Tetris players reported game-related imagery as they fell asleep. They talked about tiles falling and rotating and trying to fit blocks together. Even though they weren't new to the game, half of the expert players reported Tetris images as they fell asleep. Some novice as well as expert players reported thoughts of the game without related images. These thoughts are associated with declarative memory, which relies on the hippocampus.

Two of the five expert players dreamed of an earlier version of Tetris they had played in the past, with different colours and boxes. One subject heard music from the previous version of the game. Interestingly, the version of Tetris used for the study was silent. This shows that images during sleep onset aren't only a reactivation of recent memories. Distant memories can also make their mark.

We harbor massive amounts of information, and we constantly dip into this well of knowledge without a second thought. We climb onto a bike and pedal without thinking about how to move our legs or shift our weight. If we play Lego with kids, we might suddenly remember the castles we used to build, reliving moments from our childhood. The memory was there all along, just out of reach. Maybe it's just that we've lost the path to certain memories. Looking for a forgotten memory is like searching for a mis-shelved book in a library. If its call number doesn't map out its exact location, it's lost to us, even if it's only a shelf away.

So how did new and expert players score after seven hours of gaming across three days? The new players improved their performance considerably while the expert players, who started out with high scores, didn't improve significantly across the six gaming sessions.

Then there were the remarkable findings of the subjects with amnesia. For three of the five subjects, Tetris images appeared in their dreams. One person tried to align the shapes while another reported squares falling as they tried to put them in the right place. They generated similar vivid imagery without a properly functioning hippocampus. Even though they didn't have episodic memories of playing Tetris, they brought up implicit memories of falling colourful blocks and, in one case, playing some kind of game.[6] "They had clear Tetris imagery, and just didn't know where it was from," said Stickgold. Across all the subjects with amnesia, there was only one report of a thought about the game without an associated image. Did practicing Tetris affect their performance, even if they had no memory of it? The subjects with amnesia improved their scores over several days of gaming, just like the novice Tetris players.

How, you might wonder, did the Tetris players dream similar images? The brain is in constant recording mode, and as it sorts through information, it might find something that could have gone better. "A fruitful topic for further work," Stickgold explained. This is what makes it important and unsettled, telling us it would be useful to give it more attention. It seems the same phenomenon happened for subjects without a working hippocampus.

This brings us back to the Alpine Racer II game. In one of Stickgold's studies, subjects played the downhill skiing game. After they spent hours navigating the difficult course, subjects experienced similar images at sleep onset. In fact, Alpine Racer II had a "profoundly strong influence" on people's sensory images as they drifted off to sleep.[7] The real energy came when their players crashed and tumbled head over heels or narrowly missed falling. These were important moments. Unfinished business that they needed to work through. While speeding straight down the hill was probably exhilarating at the time, it wouldn't have been much help to dream about it. People didn't dream of the screen framing the action or their feet planted in the foot pedals or their fingers around the hand grips. They were in the game, living it.

The Lingering Scent of Roses

AS RESEARCHERS CONTINUE TO investigate the relationship between memory and sleep, many studies point to the important role of slow-wave sleep in memory consolidation, including declarative memories, which combine the factual information of semantic memories with the personal experience of episodic memories. For example, my declarative memory of Heathrow Airport taps into my knowledge that it's the UK's largest airport and combines this with my personal experience of trying to distract our son while waiting in Heathrow's long customs line. Many studies show that subjects perform better on declarative tasks like word paring after slow-wave sleep, compared to REM sleep or staying awake for the same amount of time.

In recent years, scientists have investigated Targeted Memory Reactivation (TMR) in sleep and memory studies. This technique is designed to boost memory consolidation during sleep. Here's how it works. Let's say you are learning a new task, say pairing known and unknown words. While you take in this new information, you are exposed to sensory stimuli such as sound or smell. Later on during sleep, the stimuli are replayed to reactivate the associated memory. Then the targeted memory is tested once the person is awake. The idea is to focus the sleeping brain on a particular memory to strengthen and integrate it during sleep. While TMR can be used in different sleep stages, it seems to work well in slow-wave sleep, which is thought to enhance certain memories. Many studies have tested the effects of TMR on memory tasks like word paring, word associations, and spatial learning.

In a 2007 study, Björn Rasch used an odour to flag a memory during slow-wave sleep. Subjects were exposed to the smell of roses during a spatial learning task, which uses the hippocampus, memorizing the location of card pairs on a five-by-six grid. (Imagine the kids' card-matching game Memory, where you flip over cards to make pairs, remembering the location of objects as you go.) During slow-wave sleep, one group of subjects was exposed to the scent while another group was not. A person's performance on the task improved only when they were exposed to the sweet smell of roses during slow-wave sleep. The card pairing didn't improve when the odour was emitted during REM sleep.

For another experiment in the study, the scent was introduced while subjects did a procedural task, which generally relies less on the hippocampus. They learned a finger tapping sequence on a keyboard and focused on speed and accuracy of the five-element sequence. The speed of tapping improved after sleep. Yet the learning was not enhanced for the subjects exposed to the scent during slow-wave sleep. Unlike the subjects who learned card-pairing, using their declarative memory, the performance of subjects doing the procedural task of finger tapping was unaffected by the odour. The sleep, not the scent, seemed to have an effect. When the odour was reintroduced during REM sleep, this did not affect people's performance on the finger-tapping exercise.[8]

A couple of years later, another TMR study paired sound with spatial learning of objects on a grid. Subjects learned the location of different objects, which were paired with corresponding sounds. For example, when they learned the location of a cat on their computer screen, they heard a meowing sound. Then during slow-wave sleep, subjects were re-exposed to the associated sounds for half of the fifty learned objects. When they awoke, subjects were tested on the location of objects. They were more accurate on the placement of objects with sounds that were played during NREM sleep. An additional group of participants who were exposed to associated sounds while they were awake showed no difference in memory performance.[9]

A recent study by Xiaoqing Hu used sound to target social biases during sleep. Subjects completed an implicit association test that linked faces with words to see how much gender was associated with certain subjects and if race was associated with words categorized as good or bad. For example, a white woman's face was paired with "math" while a Black man's face was paired with "sunshine." They performed counter-bias training for gender and race with associated sounds. Subjects were re-exposed to the sound for counter-gender bias and for counter-racial bias during slow-wave sleep. Racial and gender bias diminished among subjects exposed to the associated sounds during sleep, and this effect continued a week later. When sounds weren't played during sleep, the counter-bias training tended to diminish and people returned to their original biases.[10]

These findings raise the possibility of using TMR to improve well-being. What if we could target positive memories, reactivating them during sleep? Emotional memories often appear in our dreams. It's thought that sleep helps us process emotions and come to grips with the upsets and difficulties in life. Could TMR strengthen and integrate positive memories into our existing library of memories, improving our well-being?

We spend a large portion of our waking hours mind-wandering from one memory to another as a montage of thoughts floats around our heads. It's thought that a similar process happens when we're asleep. Our minds drift from one idea or situation to the next. Out of touch with the world around us, we focus on internally generated spontaneous thoughts and experiences. Often, we dream about our worries and preoccupations, focusing on what's emotional or important to us. Different areas of the brain are busy processing information. With TMR, "we think it's sort of hijacking a mechanism that's working anyway," explained American cognitive neuroscientist Ken Paller. The cortex is busy processing information and making predictions all the time. "By using the sensory channels, we push it in one direction or another, which is why I think we can push it in a positive direction to enhance well-being, regardless of your dreaming."

In Paller's Cognitive Neuroscience Laboratory at Northwestern University, they are investigating the possibility of cultivating calm sleep, linking sounds or other stimuli with a calming experience to reactivate a peaceful state of mind during sleep. They're working on strategies that change brain activity for the better, said Paller, and sound seems to be a good way to do this. The bidirectional relationship between sleep and well-being is an emerging area of study, and I'm excited to follow its progress.

Dreaming Outside the Box

THE MOST PRECIOUS ACTIVITY the human brain performs is creating meaning, explained Stickgold, who pointed out that this is far more difficult than simply memorizing facts. Information becomes meaningful when we give it context, both in the moment and in relation to the past. To understand the power of context, Stickgold offered a hypothetical example. Imagine you went out with a friend, and during dinner you had a fight. Your own personal history and the times you had with this friend got wrapped up in the meaning you gave that fight. Maybe you created meaning based on past fights with other people. Or it could be that you and this particular friend often had arguments. So a disagreement over the kind of pizza to order became something bigger, a part of your complicated history together. Then there's our personal history that we carry with us, shaping our perception of situations, which others might have no idea about. It could seem that we're overreacting if people aren't given context. Meaning is gained when you situate an experience within the thoughts, emotions, and events—the context— of your life.

The dreaming brain has a natural ability to form connections between recent and distant memories that we might overlook during the day. It seems that in dreams, we create meaning through context. A recent dream model by Stickgold and Antonio Zadra proposes a different kind of memory processing during sleep.

NEXTUP, which stands for network exploration to understand possibilities, looks at the abstract associations we make between memories while we sleep. We take recent memories and connect them with experiences and knowledge from our past. By linking them in a dream, we learn by exploring their abstract or weak associations. "Of course it's not finding answers. It's finding possibilities," explained Stickgold. I imagine dreams as our very own writer's room where we let our stream of consciousness try out whatever thought comes to mind while we're free from our daytime linear thinking. Dreams provide this open and creative space to adopt different perspectives and brainstorm new ideas. "It's the equivalent to our brain opening all these drawers in our semantic knowledge and in our autobiographical memories and everything else we've accumulated to that point and going, does it fit in here and here and here?" said Zadra.[11]

A possible function of dreaming is to find those memories that are tucked away in our brains, which might turn out to be useful if we happen to notice them. There are all sorts of ways that memories can be useful or important to us. Yet some information might turn out to have no use at all, and we can just forget about it. By connecting what we recently learned or experienced with what we already know, we give this new information deeper meaning. It's the context that provides meaning within our lives. It seems that we make different associations at different times in the night.

During sleep onset, we line up information for processing later in the night, specifically thoughts that are important and unsettled and tug at our attention. Food for thought, or dreams. During Stage 2 of the sleep cycle, our brain searches for closer associations, relatively recent thoughts or experiences that might be of value, explained Stickgold. This aligns with previous studies that found dreams during early NREM periods tend to involve relatively recent episodic memories. You might dream about a flying saucer because you went out for pizza and watched the chef fling the dough into the air.

During REM sleep, the dreaming brain finds more distant and abstract associations. This final stage of the sleep cycle is characterized by bizarre, vivid, and emotional dreams, which no doubt are filled with strange and abstract associations of memories. Dreams during REM sleep tend to relate back to ill-defined times and semantic memory, said Stickgold. As we progress through the night, our REM periods become longer and we extend our exploration for abstract associations. So if we dreamt about a flying saucer during NREM sleep because we'd had delicious pizza that day, a dream during REM might be about finding the perfect venue for an upcoming party. In this possible REM dream, we explore different possibilities that come from the abstract association of having found the best pizza place.

For me, one of the confounding questions around dreams is why we dream about distant memories at certain times. How does the dreaming brain pull open drawer after drawer of memories and choose that one moment from decades ago? Or maybe take a distant memory and rescript it in a completely new way. What made me dream about my drafty university apartment last night, of all nights? And why couldn't I lock our back door? A simple answer is that my old roommate texted me before bed. Could my dreaming brain have landed on this memory through more abstract associations? Maybe it related to my son heading off to university. We don't need to remember our dreams to benefit from this creative memory processing. In the case of searching for the perfect party venue, we might wake up thinking of some new possibilities without remembering what we dreamt. According to Portuguese neuroscientist Antonio Damasio, one of the main functions of consciousness is that it lets us construct narratives, and by creating stories, we learn from the past and imagine our future.

During the altered state of dreaming, as we test out new scenarios and contextualize them within our existing library of experiences, emotions, and knowledge, we're given different perspectives on our current situation as well as our future. A dream about eating the best pizza might not seem like an earth-shattering, philosophically important event. But what if we shifted our perspective. Turned the table, so to speak, and considered that the dream might be about the person who sat across from us. Maybe it gave us a fresh outlook on the person and our relationship with them.

Dreams continue to do their work into the next day. That is, if we choose to pay attention to them. They might spark new ideas or sharpen our focus on our current worries and preoccupations. A kind of added bonus that's beyond their biological function. Could the real value of dreams be found in their intrinsic connection to our waking lives?

Chapter Eight

LIFE UNFILTERED

IN 1933, THREE DAYS AFTER HITLER CAME TO POWER, THIRD Reich propagandist Joseph Goebbels walked into a factory and lined up the workers in two rows. The factory owner, Herr S., stood in between the rows of workers as he struggled to raise his arm in the Nazi salute. For half an hour, Herr S. lifted his arm, inch by inch, while Goebbels watched, expressionless. Finally, Herr S. extended his arm. Palm down. Fingers together. "I don't want your salute," declared Goebbels who turned to leave. Herr S. stood in front of his fellow social democrats, arm raised in salute to Hitler. To keep from collapsing, the sixty-year-old man fixed his gaze on Goebbels's foot, which was twisted inward from a congenital condition, as the politician limped out of sight.

Suddenly, Herr S. bolted awake. It was all a dream. Yet his feelings of alienation and loss of identity under Nazi rule continued to shape his days and nights. The man was tormented by his recurrent factory dream that transformed with new, mortifying details. One night, sweat ran down his face as he stood in front of Goebbels. In another dream, Herr S. broke his backbone, struggling to lift his arm into the Nazi salute.

Around the same time, Jewish journalist Charlotte Beradt was living in Berlin. She and her husband, Heinz Pol, were detained during mass arrests of communists. Beradt and Pol were released. Yet Beradt was barred from publishing her writing. So she recorded Herr S.'s dreams in secret. Then she used the factory worker's dreams to encourage others to share their own dream stories as she investigated the Third Reich's expansion into the private inner realm of dreams.

Beradt collected and analyzed people's dreams that were influenced by the Nazi regime. From 1933 to 1939, Beradt collected three hundred dreams, including those of an aunt, a neighbour, the milkman, and a dressmaker. Many people were afraid to talk about their dreams, which led some to dream that they were forbidden to even dream.

Beradt created a collective dream journal of German people, revealing how freedom of thought was out of reach, even in their dreams. Their dreams were "dictated to them by dictatorship,"[2] wrote Beradt. A woman dreamt that posters had replaced street signs on every corner, announcing forbidden words. The first was "lord," which the woman dreamt in English, just to be safe, and the last word was "I," which reflected the loss of identity under the totalitarian rule. In another dream, the woman found herself sitting in a box at the opera, watching *The Magic Flute*. She wore a new gown and had beautifully styled hair that was admired by people in the audience. When an actor said she must be the devil, police officers surrounded her. A machine registered her thinking of Hitler when the word "devil" was uttered.

Many dreams in Beradt's collection reflected the feeling of turmoil and uncertainty as Nazi regulations imposed order in often nonsensical ways. A forty-five-year-old doctor dreamt of relaxing on his couch after seeing his last patient of the day. Without warning, the walls of his apartment disappeared. He looked around to discover that all of the apartments were void of walls. Then a loudspeaker announced the abolition of walls.

There were book burnings and mass home searches as the Nazis looked for political subversives. Beradt hid her transcripts in the bindings of books that she dispersed throughout her large library. Later on, she mailed the dream stories as letters to friends abroad.

In 1939, Beradt fled Germany. She landed in New York as a refugee with her second husband, Martin Beradt. It would be years before the transcripts of her fellow Germans' dream stories were returned to her. In 1966, *Das Dritte Reich des Traums* (The Third Reich of Dreams) was published in Germany. In 1968, the English translation was released. After more than forty years out of print, this important title in the canon of Holocaust literature was republished in 2025.

Beradt offers a rare perspective on the workings of the German mind during Hitler's reign. German people relinquished free expression, even in their dreams. The book illustrates in painful detail how our dreams reflect our waking preoccupations and fears. We cannot hide, even from ourselves. Beradt noted that the dreams seemed almost conscious and free of façade as "an echo of daily life reverberates with frightening loudness."[3]

Worlds Collide

IT WAS AMERICAN PSYCHOLOGIST Calvin S. Hall who formalized the idea that dreams reflect our everyday existence, with his "continuity hypothesis," which described the continuity between dreams and waking life. We don't just dream about our experiences. We dream of our thoughts and feelings about our lives, including our relationships and any concerns weighing on our minds. For the most part, dreams are coherent depictions of life. They play out endless scenarios of what could happen—or what we hope or dread will happen. While most dreams aren't exact replays of waking events, one well-known study found that more than half of dream reports include at least one element from waking experiences.[4]

Hall conducted content analysis of dreams, gaining insights into individuals, groups of people, and humanity overall. In the 1940s, Hall collected thousands of anonymous dream reports from college students. He created categories to quantify common dream elements and study patterns in content across series of dreams. This allowed Hall to identify and compare dream features among groups of people.

Hall and psychologist Robert Van de Castle developed the Hall/Van de Castle (HVDC) dream coding system, which became the standard dream analysis tool and is still used today. Anyone can code and analyze their dreams with the HVDC system, which is available online.

The HVDC system scores dream content by classifying and counting dream elements using many distinct categories: characters, activities, success and failure, misfortune and good fortune, emotions, settings, objects, descriptive elements, and social interactions, which are divided into aggression, friendliness, and sexuality. Three categories you might want to focus on are characters, social interactions, and emotions. Characters include people from waking life, animals, and mythical beings. Since we are usually the protagonist of our dreams, we do not include ourselves as a character to be coded. Characters are classified by their identity. The character could be a relative, someone known to the dreamer, a prominent person, or someone identified by their occupation like a police officer or doctor. Social interactions include aggressive acts like being chased or hurt, friendly acts like petting a dog or smiling, and sexual interactions. Dream emotions are classified as feelings like anger, apprehension, sadness, confusion, or happiness.

Once a dream has been scored, the results can be compared to a set of norms created by Hall and Van de Castle. The psychologists compiled five dream reports from one hundred men and one hundred women at Case Western University, creating norms for comparative analysis. Are you curious to know if your dreams are overly aggressive? The Hall/Van de Castle norms found that about 80 percent of women's and men's dreams had dreamer-involved aggression. Do you wonder if you dream about sex more than others? Tally up your sex-related dream elements and compare them to the norms, which found sexuality present in 12 percent of men's dreams and 4 percent of women's dreams.[5]

If we analyze common dream elements, this can highlight which waking activities, thoughts, and concerns take centre stage in our dreams. Do certain people or experiences continue to make an appearance in our nightly stories? If we look at a series of dreams, is there a particular concern or thought that is a central theme? This might offer different perspectives on what is happening as well as what we *think* is happening in our lives.

Hall believed that dreams are the "embodiment of thoughts." He explained, "That which is invisible, namely a conception, becomes visible when it is transformed into a dream image."[6] In dreams, we are given a candid view of how we see ourselves at a certain point in time. Our conceptions, along with our dreams, change throughout our lives as we amass experiences, gain knowledge, and connect with new people.

When I was twenty, I made the long trek from Toronto to the Yukon, then caught the weekly bus to the old gold rush town of Atlin, British Columbia, for a two-week writers' retreat. We workshopped ideas, then strapped ice cleats onto our mountain boots, hiked icy trails, and camped under the midnight sun, darkness never descending. It was difficult and uncomfortable and absolutely magical. When I returned home, I dreamt of Sky, the white husky who guarded our tent, and hiking Ruby Mountain with my newfound friends. There's a picture of four of us. I don't know where it is anymore, but sometimes I dream of the day it was taken.

While the HVDC coding system classifies dream elements, it's up to us to contextualize the findings within our waking lives. We are our own dream interpreter, analyzing our dreams and the feelings they evoke. We are also the decoder of our dreams, mapping experiences from our waking lives. We get to decide what our dreams might be trying to tell us and what calls for our attention. We can think about the people, emotions, or situations that keep popping up, and ask ourselves why. We can compare our waking self-image to how we portray ourselves in dreams. In my recurrent dream about that summer in northern B.C., the details often change, like whether we're playing cards in front of our tent or sharing stories under an earthy orange sky. The image of my carefree younger self remains the same. Using the HVDC system, I notice there are many friendly social interactions in my Atlin dreams. We're often smiling and leaning into each other, unable to contain our laughter. The serious stuff of mid-life—all the grown-up responsibilities and worries—is yet to happen.

Hall believed that dreams call attention to our waking issues and concerns. Often a dream "illuminates a major conflict like a spotlight shooting its beam into the darkness," he wrote in the late 1940s. Hall found that there is often a main conflict. This tension can shape a series of dreams, with each dream as its own piece of the same puzzle. "The individual dreams are fitted together by testing one inference after another until an interlocking, coherent, organized, and meaningful appraisal is obtained."[7]

This makes me think of a series of stressful dreams I've been having about work, which seem to focus on responsibility and competency. In one dream, there was a horrible accident on the highway that prevented me from getting to work. When I finally made it to the office, my desk had vanished. In another dream, I was on stage, presenting in front of a large audience. I saw people's confused faces and looked behind me to find a blank screen. All my slides had been erased.

Then one night, I dreamt of camping in Algonquin Park, a large, forested area in northern Ontario. I imagined the tall trees swaying and creaking in the wind and the white beam of my flashlight bobbing through the darkness, guiding me and my daughter to the rest station. Suddenly I was back in Atlin, B.C., playing cards around a tree stump that was our improvised card table. At first glance, my dream about camping and those carefree summer weeks in northern B.C. had nothing to do with my work dreams. But maybe the stark contrast was the point. Camping has always been the calm within the storm of daily responsibilities and worries. I hadn't given my camping dreams much thought. Now they seemed like a vacation from my work dreams.

When I think about it, the worries showing up in my dreams aren't a complete surprise. Hall found that most of us are aware of the conflicts and concerns that appear in our dreams. He believed these concerns are transparent rather than disguised, as Freud contended. When collecting people's dreams, Hall would ask for their interpretation. He found that people were good at interpreting their own dreams without knowing about Freudian symbolism. "Why should one bother to deceive oneself by dreaming in symbols when they can be translated so readily by the dreamer himself?" asked Hall.[8] Trying to suppress our worries isn't the solution. In fact, thought suppression seems to make unwanted thoughts rebound in our dreams.

Adjusting Our Lens

HALL'S RIGOROUS STUDY OF dream content revealed that we can learn a lot from our dreams. Across several decades of dream research, he amassed more than fifty thousand dream reports from college students, children, avid dreamers, and adults from different places around the world. One of Hall's key insights was that our dreams reflect not only our waking experiences, but also what we think and feel about these experiences. Think about Herr S. raising his right arm in the Nazi salute. The German factory owner didn't simply dream about lifting his right arm, inch by inch. He dreamt of his humiliation in front of his workers. With each new take on the same recurrent dream, Herr S.'s experience intensified. As sweat ran down his face, reminding him of tears, he stood there, powerless, in front of the factory workers whose faces showed "absolute emptiness."[9]

Hall had an interesting case in which he analyzed the dreams of an engineer known as Karl. The man was in his early thirties and sent Hall more than a thousand dream reports. When Hall analyzed the reports, Karl offered some clarifications that gave Hall a different perspective on his analysis. Karl reported a number of aggressive dreams involving his father. Hall inferred that Karl was an angry person who sometimes got into fights. Karl explained that he didn't fight with people and considered himself friendly and peaceful. It turned out that the aggressive interactions were related to his father, not his overall demeanor. In another instance, Karl reported many dreams about football, which led Hall to believe that he was an avid player. While he hadn't thrown a football in years, Karl still thought about the sport and even pictured being a professional footballer. It was his thoughts and feelings about his life that shaped these dreams. As social psychologist G. William Domhoff points out, Karl's football dreams are an example of "unfinished business" that appears in dreams.[10] We often dream of unresolved issues, working through what's important to us.

Domhoff and Adam Schneider created DreamBank, a free online database of more than twenty thousand dreams collected over many decades from dreamers aged seven to seventy-four. The anonymized dream reports are from different sources, with many dreams coded using the HVDC system. Anyone can search this fascinating collection of dreams at DreamBank.net and conduct their own dream analysis. Choose an element that appears regularly in your dreams and search the database to see if it's common or unusual. You can learn what university students in Cleveland, Ohio, dreamt about in the 1940s, read the war dreams of a Vietnam veteran, or see what kids in Germany dreamt about in the early 1990s. Or you can delve into the dream world of a widower who recorded more than one hundred and forty dreams of his late wife.

Domhoff analyzed a long series of dreams from a widower known as Ed. For more than two decades, Ed recorded dreams about his late wife, Mary, who died of ovarian cancer in her mid-fifties. To cope with his sorrow and isolation, Ed started keeping a dream journal. "So when I had a dream in which Mary appeared, it was like a precious moment of being with her again. I wanted to capture that fleeting moment and hold onto it forever."[11] Before this, he'd had little interest in his dreams.

Ed had many different types of dreams about Mary. He often dreamt of her sick and dying, which reflected his thoughts of his wife's fatal illness. There were "back-to-life dreams" in which Mary returned and "reassurance dreams" where Mary tried to help her husband cope with her death. It was one of these dreams that touched Ed so deeply it compelled him to keep a dream journal. Ed described it as a scene played out on TV with a voice-over of Mary saying, "I want you to be happy, Ed."[12]

Psychologist David Foulkes studied thousands of dreams of children, teenagers, and adults and found that dreams are "credible world analogs" or "simulations" of waking experiences.[13] Teenagers often dream of going shopping, arguing with their parents, or playing sports. Using episodic memories and our knowledge of the world, dreams create lifelike situations, often involving people we know.

Deep Thoughts of the Dreaming Brain

IN RECENT YEARS, DREAM researchers have studied the continuity hypothesis beyond dream content to examine the thought processes that create our dreams. Even though dreams are often bizarre and nonsensical, the thought processes that make these wild works of fiction might be quite rational. In dreams, we seem to use some high-level thinking similar to what we use throughout the day to plan, make decisions, and form conclusions. In 2007, Richard N. Wolman and Miloslava Kozmová demonstrated that many categories of rational thought processes are involved in dreaming.

Wolman and Kozmová studied forty dreams from subjects with varied backgrounds including a stockbroker, lawyer, supervisor of a psychiatric ward, and three administrative assistants. The researchers discovered that analytical thinking was the most common type of rational thought process. Analytical thinking incorporates reasoning, comparing, and reflecting. One person reported, "I express amazement as I had expected a simple civil proceeding and have no knowledge of a criminal case."[14] Perceptual thought was the second most common category of rational thought. This involves seeing, hearing, touching, and smelling. Another person reported, "I saw that everyone in the room was crouched down on the floor using tables and chairs as shields." The third most popular type of rational thought was memory and awareness of time. This involves remembering, recalling, and recognizing people, places, and events from the waking world. One subject recognized a map of Europe in their dream. Wolman and Kozmová showed the continuity of rational and complex thought processes from waking life.

In 2011, Tracey Kahan and Stephen LaBerge tested the hypothesis that the dreaming mind is very similar to the waking mind. They found that subjects reported high-level cognitive skills that are characteristic of waking thought, including focused attention, planning, decision-making, and reflective awareness. Kahan and LaBerge concluded that "high-order cognition is much more common in dreams than has been assumed, so any theory of dreaming that does not take this into account is out-of-date."[15]

For dream researcher Michael Schredl, dreaming is a subjective experience during sleep that we believe to be real. When I spoke with Schredl, he pointed out how our dreaming brain operates in a different mode. To help me understand how this works, he compared it to drinking a bottle of wine, which changes the brain's physiology. "It's also changing the way you experience things. And that's the same if you compare daydreaming, NREM, and REM dreaming," he explained.

Dreaming offers another dimension of experience, one that we are easily convinced is real because we are in a different brain state. "Dreams are exaggerations of waking life feelings," said Schredl, who has been researching dreams for more than three decades. A falling dream might amplify our waking feelings of helplessness. Maybe we are unsure about a job or our current situation in life.

Dreams, like waking experiences, can affect our thoughts and emotions, even our behaviour. In one study, Schredl and Anja S. Göritz found that 37 percent of people contacted someone after dreaming about them.[16] Some dreams are so impactful that they have a transformative effect on people's lives. These powerful "big dreams," as Carl Jung called them, can inspire major decisions or life changes.

If dreams are as real to us as waking experiences, how might they affect our identity and sense of self? Our identity is our own creation. We construct stories about ourselves. We take our interpretations of the world and hold onto memories that help us decide who we think we are. As we amass new experiences, our memories are revised and sometimes replaced, and we are forever editing our perception of ourselves.

Our impressions have the power to shape who we are, in both our dreaming and waking lives. When we fall asleep, we disconnect from the day's obligations and distractions. The dreaming mind is free from the filters of waking life, released from the perceptions, assumptions, and expectations that shape our self-image. In dreams, we are given insights into who we think we are and wish to become. How do we see ourselves in our dreams? Maybe during the day, we appear calm and self-assured while our uncertainties reveal themselves in our dreams. It could be said that our dream thoughts are as much a part of us as our waking preoccupations. When we examine them in the morning, they may seem at odds with who we think we are.

As sleep medicine pioneer William Dement pointed out, dreaming is the "nightly disembodiment of the self" that lets us time travel or visit otherworldly dimensions.[17] Dement asked, "Can it be the same self whose hand reaches out to hush the alarm clock, who yawns and stretches, waking to the cold light of day?" If we look at dreams along our continuum of experience, as happening in an altered state of consciousness, then it makes sense that our dreams help shape us. As for the strange and puzzling dream stories, we can read them as fictions that we've written while our brain is working in a different mode. As Walt Whitman famously said, "Do I contradict myself? / Very well then I contradict myself, / (I am large, I contain multitudes.)"[18] In dreams and waking life, we are an abundance of truths and contradictions to many people, including ourselves.

Same Old Story, Different Dream

WHILE THE DETAILS OF our dreams are as unique as each of us, researchers have discovered several common emotions, conflicts, and concerns that appear regularly in dreams. As Hall discovered, our lives may be very different, yet we tend to be preoccupied by similar worries, which play out in our dreams.

In 2009, American dream researcher and author Kelly Bulkeley launched a searchable catalogue of dreams, the Sleep and Dream Database (SDDB). It's a diverse collection of more than forty thousand dreams that is compiled from many sources. The database spans dream reports from the second century to the present, including the collection of Roman orator Aelius Aristides. You can read about other people's dreams, from around the globe, or study your own.

Analyzing thousands of dreams, Bulkeley found striking consistency in the appearance of certain dream elements and emotions. Across dreams from different countries, times in history, and ages of dreamers, Bulkeley found more reports of fear than happiness, more dreams reflecting wonder and confusion than anger, while sadness was the least reported emotion. "That does not look like a mish-mash of random content; it starts to look like a fairly stable pattern of emotional expression in dreaming," noted Bulkeley.[19] Over the years, many studies have found that bad dreams are quite common, with many lab and home studies reporting that more than two-thirds of dreams are negative.[20] This isn't necessarily a bad thing. It turns out that some negative dreams help us process difficult emotions.

There are many common themes that show up in dreams. This includes work dreams where we play out stresses and preoccupations around work in different ways. The variations are endless. Some might imagine being late or unable to get to the office while others might dream of a disastrous presentation or altercation with a colleague. We spend most of our time either working or thinking about work, so it makes sense that our dreaming minds keep returning to the office. It seems unfair to have to work even in our dreams. But the dreaming brain's hard work has many benefits.

Personal relationships also tend to show up, especially at times of crisis and change. Flying dreams are common, which can be empowering for people who are afraid of heights. Another common topic is teeth, with people dreaming about a bad toothache or their teeth falling out. Others imagine driving a car that is out of control. As with the stories we tell during the day, the details of our dream stories are all our own. Maybe we imagine our brakes failing. Or maybe our steering wheel locks and we head straight for the guardrail of a highway.

Many athletes have upsetting dreams before a big game or competition, while students may have bad dreams the night before an exam. Interestingly, exam dreams can pop up years after we've graduated. One idea is that we explore the theme of competency by dreaming that we're being tested. It can be interesting to connect what's happening in our waking lives with recurrent dreams. Are there certain emotions, settings, or characters that keep popping up across a series of dreams? How could it relate to waking life, and how do we feel about it? There are many tools and techniques we can use to better understand what's happening in our dreams.

Then there are the dreams at pivotal points in your life that can cause a seismic shift in your thinking. Researchers have found that many of us dream of divorce, illness, and loss. Through the widower Ed's dreams, we learned how losing a loved one can shape our dreams. Pregnancy is another life-changing moment that I discovered has the power to influence our dreams.

"Emotional Ultrasound"

IT'S THE MIDDLE OF the night, and I'm lying on a hospital gurney parked in a busy corridor of an emergency room. My body feels lost under a thin green sheet, which I grasp with tight fists. My bare toes ache from the cold wind whipping through the sliding glass doors, and goose bumps shoot up along my arms. Suddenly I'm blanketed by my duvet from home, but it's snatched away as quickly as it appears. A nurse says I mustn't get too warm or comfortable before the surgery.

I hoist myself up to survey the situation, but several pairs of hands clamp down on my shoulders, pushing me back down onto unforgiving steel. Masked faces hover overhead, mumbling to one another. I wish I knew what they were saying. With a forceful push of the gurney, we head down the corridor. The faces of other patients flash beside me, as if I were staring out the window of a speeding car. The gurney crashes through swinging doors into an operating room, stopping under a blinding light. I listen to the clink of metal as a gloved hand lays out a row of surgical instruments. I am hooked up to a heart-rate monitor that emits high-pitched, staccato beats.

A comforting hand squeezes my arm, and a familiar voice says, "Don't worry. You're going to be fine." It's my husband in hospital scrubs. Squinting at the other masked faces, I begin to recognize people's eyes, including those of my mother, who says, "You're here for open-heart surgery," as she adjusts her gloves. "Nothing to worry about." A friend says they'll be performing the surgery. I'm quietly freaking out. But I don't want to hurt anyone's feelings so I just lie there, watching the scalpel descend toward my chest. Just as it's about to pierce my skin, the scene changes, and I'm alone in the OR, doubled over with labor pains.

The cavernous room reminds me of my high school gymnasium, echoing every wail and scream. Sweat drips from my blotchy red face. How can I deliver my baby on my own? Through the pain, I feel a burst of joy as I look down and wiggle my toes, which are now warm inside my favorite pair of socks. The double doors fan open, and I catch a glimpse of my husband sitting in our living room. I scream for his attention, but the doors swing closed before he can hear me. I keep staring at the closed doors until they open again. I yell his name, and he looks up, shocked to see me lying there. He runs into the delivery room with a handful of garden tools. "What do you need?" he asks. I bolt awake to find myself lying in bed beside him.

It's remarkable how this dream has stayed with me for nearly two decades. Alexander was our first child, and during the day, I was preoccupied with all the planning and preparations that parenthood brings. It's when I lay down at night that my worries took over. Was I qualified to be a mother? What were my credentials? A yearning to have a child and a grade seven babysitting course at the YMCA? With each passing day, my sense of self seemed to shift, and in nine months, I'd be forever changed. As dream researcher Rosalind Cartwright explained, "In sleep, the process of becoming persists. Matters that we usually keep in the background while awake—our feelings about what's happening in our lives—claim the foreground in sleep."[21]

I wasn't alone in my fears. Scientists have found that pregnant women, particularly those carrying their firstborn, are often haunted by emotionally charged dreams. At a time of transformation, expectant mothers are acutely aware of their baby's dependence on them for survival. They question their readiness for parenthood and become overwhelmed by the prospect of labor and delivery as well as by changes in self-image. American psychologist Alan Siegel sees dreams as an "emotional ultrasound" during pregnancy. For expectant mothers, dreams offer a glimpse into how they are responding to their changing identity, marriage, and close relationships while their attachment to their unborn child grows.[22]

Disturbing as these anxiety-ridden dreams may be, researchers have found that they do serve a purpose. Carolyn Winget and Frederic Kapp found that pregnant women who had anxiety-ridden dreams were likelier to have shorter labors. They studied the dreams of seventy women during the third trimester of their first pregnancy. Reviewing their dream reports, Winget and Kapp found a significant relationship between the emotions in the women's dreams and the length of delivery. More than 80 percent of women who delivered in less than ten hours had had anxiety dreams. Of the women who took more than twenty hours to deliver, only 25 percent had anxiety-ridden dreams. The findings supported the idea that dreams help us master or come to grips with an "anticipated stress" in our waking lives. The authors noted that dreams are a kind of "problem-solving mechanism" for expectant mothers to prepare for their major life change.[23]

Distressing dreams don't always end after a baby is born. In one study, Tore Nielsen and Tyna Paquette studied the dreams of postpartum and pregnant women. They found that about 73 percent of new mothers dreamt their newborns were in danger, lost, or hurt. Approximately 41 percent of the new mothers reported lingering anxiety, while 60 percent reported checking on their baby following such a dream. Many postpartum women dreamt of their baby getting lost or suffocated in bed, causing them to search for the newborn under the covers. Even when these new mothers realized the baby wasn't in their bed, many were compelled to check that their baby was safely asleep. The researchers called this common episode the baby-in-bed (BIB) nightmare pattern. These dreams may reflect a mother's "state of maternal vigilance; they may even serve a functional role in her infant caregiving," explained the researchers.

Many pregnant subjects experienced traumatic dreams. A month before her delivery, one woman dreamt of a foot coming out of her pregnant stomach. "I tried to get it back inside when the other one came out and then the head too, but on the top of the belly," reported the expectant mother. "I told my husband that we had to hurry to the hospital because the baby wasn't ready to come out yet and, if it did, it would die."[24]

This happens as new and expectant mothers form attachments with their baby. This includes picturing what life will be like as a parent. Impressions of their new life are carried into their dreams, which illuminate their worries and uncertainties. "Our dreams review and revise our concept of who we are, and they rehearse where we are going," explained Rosalind Cartwright. "Moreover, in times of trouble, if they function as they should, dreams provide a fourth R, a mechanism for repair."[25] For decades, Cartwright studied the dreams of people during times of personal crisis. Cartwright's work reflected the possible function of dreaming to help us process and regulate emotions.

If we tune into our dreams, we might just find new insights into ourselves and our current state of mind. There are many ways that we can use our dreams to improve our waking lives. A group of Stanford researchers have discovered that a certain kind of intense and surreal dream experience has the power to create big change in people's lives.

Chapter Nine

THE POWER OF
BIG DREAMS

THERE'S A LOCAL PARK NEAR MARE LUCAS'S HOUSE IN PALO
Alto, California, with a playground and a big open field that's perfect for
playing catch or having a game of tag as kids giggle wildly and chase one
another across the grass. In 2022, Lucas watched her two sons play with
their dog, a corgi named Moxie.

Eighteen-year-old Zane and his youngest brother ran around with their
dog while Lucas listened to her boys laughing and having fun. She tuned in
to the distinct sound of each boy's voice. Zane was a big kid, tall and muscu-
lar, with a deep voice and a booming laugh. His youngest brother had more
of a chuckle that drifted toward her. "I'm soaking in the joy and the beauty
and the laughter," said the mother of four as she described the scene to me. "I
would almost pay anything to have another one of these experiences. That's
how powerful it is." In this magical moment, Lucas was reunited with her
son Zane who died by suicide in 2017.

While Lucas was having this transformative experience, her motionless
body lay on a surgical table in an operating room (OR) at Stanford Health
Care. Lucas was having surgery for breast cancer. It was a long procedure
that lasted several hours. As the surgical team finished up, anesthesiologist
Harrison Chow observed her brain activity on the EEG. The five electrodes
along Lucas's forehead picked up activity in the prefrontal brain regions.

Our brain produces a spectrum of frequencies as we move between the heavy sedation of general anesthesia to the moment we open our eyes again. General anesthesia quiets the frontal brain regions, which are associated with high order functions like working memory and reflective abilities. As anesthesia is lightened, these frontal areas start to get noisy with activity.

With the procedure almost done, Chow began to lighten the anesthesia, which activated the prefrontal region. But not to the point where Lucas would awaken. Chow closely monitored the EEG. He was on the lookout for small, sharp spikes of brain activity, telling him that Lucas was in a specific dreamlike state that is just underneath the surface of consciousness.

Imagine an EEG as a radio that's programmed with different stations. A patient moves across many states of consciousness that appear as different patterns of brain activity on an EEG. On one end of the continuum a patient is fully awake, and moving toward the other end they are in a deep sleep–like state under general anesthesia. There are hundreds of EEG patterns, or radio stations, that anesthesiologists can tune into. On this imagined radio, picture 50 being the number to dial in for the patient to wake up.

In the OR, Chow was on the lookout for frequency 48. Gently adjusting the anesthesia, Chow dialed into the right frequency. Then he monitored the dosage of propofol to keep Lucas there. This is the dreamlike state where Lucas was reunited with her son Zane. This is the uncharted territory of anesthesia-induced dreams.

After I spoke with Lucas about her dream, I had many questions for Chow. To begin with, what are anesthesia-induced dreams? Why do these hyperreal dreams seem to happen at frequency 48? What makes these dreams so remarkable? I discovered that many of the answers depended on whom I asked. There was the scientific explanation for this powerful and intense dream experience, a kind of transcendent "big dream" that Jung talked about. Or at least what researchers know so far from clinical observations. Then there were the profound personal experiences of dreamers like Lucas. I decided to first look at the physiology of this brain state.

Chow was the ideal guide to navigate the unmapped terrain of anesthesia dreams. Over fifteen years, he has witnessed more than fifteen hundred patients have profound dream experiences when he slowly reduced anesthesia and tuned into a peaceful state during a calm, gentle awakening. He is the "chief dream architect" of the "dream team" at Stanford University that is studying this unique dreamlike state in the OR and in the lab. "I know how to make dreams," Chow told me.

The group is part of Boris Heifets's lab at Stanford. It's made up of researchers and clinicians spanning the fields of psychiatry, sleep, neuroscience, and anesthesiology. They bring diverse perspectives and expertise to explore the physiological and psychological underpinnings of this phenomenon. I met with several scientists and physicians in the group to talk about the case series that observed the anesthesia dreams of several subjects including Lucas. We talked about what we currently know about this unique kind of dream experience, its ongoing mysteries and remarkable promise as a possible treatment for different mental health conditions, specifically PTSD. This is a new and emerging area of dream research. The idea, however, was born nearly twenty years ago from observations in the OR.

When I spoke with Chow, he took me back to 2007 when he was working in private practice as a regional anesthesiologist. To reduce sedation and nausea after surgery, Chow titrated patients' anesthesia to create a slow, peaceful awakening. He would take a few extra minutes and keep patients just under the surface of consciousness. The technique seemed to wipe out post-operative nausea. Patients woke up happy and incredibly alert.

Then Chow noticed an astounding additional observation. Patients described a dream world that was more vivid than the waking world. The sun shone brighter. The ocean was an electric blue. Along vast beaches, grains of sand were magnified. It was more like a hyperreal experience than a dream. And the experience was always positive, no matter what the dream was about. Even traumatic events were somehow transformed into positive experiences.

In 2020, Chow came to Stanford University, where along with being a dream maker, he is clinical associate professor in the department of anesthesiology, perioperative and pain medicine. With an EEG in the OR, Chow began to identify brain patterns associated with this unique dreamlike state. "We're basically using our EEG like you would use an ultrasound or X-ray to visualize something specific in the brain," explained Chow. He discovered that if he dialed into frequency 48 and kept patients just below the surface of consciousness, they experienced these transformative dreams with a Hollywood ending. "If you are tuned into that frequency, the dream will turn positive within seconds to a minute," said Chow.

When Chow described these intense experiences, it made me wonder if they were actual dreams. This brought me to the question of how we define a dream. There is a tendency to think about our dreams as separate from our waking lives. Dreams are often perceived as distinct and disconnected from reality. Maybe it's their bizarre elements. Maybe it's because they often evade our memory, disappearing as soon as we crawl out of bed in the morning. Or maybe it's that we don't pay much attention to our dreams. We can get so wrapped up in the busyness of everyday life that it's easy to overlook where dreams fit in.

Yet researchers have discovered that our dream experiences are as real to us as our waking experiences.[1] They can be as impactful as events that happen during the day. We're simply thinking and experiencing on another level of consciousness while our brain is functioning in a different state. When we dream, we create an internally generated experience that transports us beyond the four walls of our bedroom.

I met with another member of the team, Pilleriin Sikka, to understand how anesthesia-induced dreams fit with this idea. Before speaking with Sikka, I hadn't given much thought to dreams during anesthesia. The few times that I've woken from anesthesia, I never considered whether my strange thoughts were in fact dreams and where they fit on the sleep-wake cycle. Sikka explained that patients under sedation have dreamlike experiences when they're out of touch with the outside world. These experiences are not isolated. "There is no sharp divide between our waking and sleep and dream experiences," explained Sikka, postdoctoral researcher in the department of anesthesiology, perioperative and pain medicine at Stanford University. Anesthesia-induced dreams are part of our continuum of experience.

Sikka has a PhD in psychology from the University of Turku, Finland.

For her thesis, she studied the emotions and moods that we experience in dreams. "We are not machines," said Sikka. "Our experiences make us who we are." This includes our dream experiences. Every night, we have access to this alternate state of consciousness. In dreams, we don't simply replay waking events. We reflect on ideas, experiences, and sometimes difficult emotions that we're struggling to process, and explore them in unique ways. Through different variations and responses, we practice, learn, and digest information and emotions in our dreams, connecting and contextualizing these experiences with our waking lives. This effect seems to be amplified with anesthesia dreams.

I learned that anesthesia dreams are a unique phenomenon that is unlike typical dreams during NREM or REM sleep. It's difficult to determine where they fit on the sleep-wake cycle. At this point, research indicates these experiences under anesthesia are dreams rather than hallucinations or a confusional state. What remains a mystery is their physiological state.

Since the 1940s, scientists have shared their observations of dreams under anesthesia. What's new is investigating whether these impactful dreams can be used therapeutically. This reimagines how we view as well as use anesthesia, which is administered to facilitate surgery. Currently, Sikka and the team at Stanford are studying anesthesia dreams in the lab, looking for biomarkers to identify the biological mechanisms of this dreamlike state.

When patients reach the frequency where they have these positive dream experiences, it's important to keep them there for at least five minutes, explained Chow. This gives them enough time to have the experience, which can be powerful in different ways. Chow recalled when a former Olympic athlete awoke from anesthesia. In his seventies, the man asked for a few extra minutes to keep practicing his hammer throw.

Often, the impactful dreams of cancer patients involve their children or family. Kelsey Newman has had four anesthesia dreams during multiple surgeries for recurrent breast cancer. In each dream, there was a problem, a solution, and a feeling of calmness and peace. When we spoke, Newman described her fourth anesthesia dream as the "ultimate resolve." In her dream, the California teacher was travelling through Europe with her son. She imagined him as a teenager, a few years older than his actual age. Newman was on tour for a book she had written about her cancer journey. She had beaten cancer, and her son was by her side. "It was just beautiful and there was this independence with my son and the journey of it," she told me. "It was almost like it had already happened." Often with ordinary dreams, things don't make sense or seem strange. "This was real. Like it was real life," she said.

A sense of calmness and peace has stayed with Newman since she awoke from her dream after surgery in March 2024. "I don't know how I'm going to beat this. I mean I am still dealing with it," Newman told me. The vivid dream has given her hope. She described it as a premonition. "A look into the future," said Newman, when she was healthy and her son was right there with her.

Talking to patients who've experienced these dreams and scientists who study the phenomenon, I discovered a distinguishing feature of anesthesia dreams. A characteristic that makes them so remarkable, even beyond their unwavering positivity, is the impact of the experience, which can be deeply personal and life-changing. I learned how an experience that takes only minutes can leave a significant and lasting impression on people's lives.

Big Dreams

ANESTHESIA-INDUCED DREAMS ARE A kind of impactful dream, a powerful dream experience that influences a person's waking thoughts and emotions. Psychologist and researcher Don Kuiken has studied impactful dreams for decades. In the 1990s, Kuiken identified three types of impactful dreams: nightmares, existential dreams, and transcendent dreams. Nightmares have vivid, intense images and overwhelming distress for the dreamer, who often tries to escape from harm and wakes up, gripped by fear. Existential dreams feature vivid images, contrasting light and darkness, separation, loss, and fatigue, with the dreamer waking up to a feeling of profound sadness. Transcendent dreams have vivid images as well, yet these are often magical, featuring light and warmth, and the dreamer awakens with a feeling of awe and ecstasy. What sets impactful dreams apart from everyday dreams is how real the dream images seem to the dreamer and the intense effect that stays with them long after they've awakened.[2]

The more I learned about anesthesia dreams, the more I wondered how one dream can have the power to change your life. I discovered a couple of ways to understand how these unique dreams make their mark. Think of an experience that changed the tenor, the rhythm, even the progression of your life. Maybe you got married or had a child. Or maybe you survived a near-death experience. Big life events have the power to create big change. I found that these dream experiences can be just as powerful, and unlike ordinary dreams that are often negative, their power lies in their positivity.

It's natural to prioritize waking experiences over dreams. In speaking with patients like Newman and Lucas, I found that dreams can provide some of life's most memorable moments. Our dream stories are part of our catalogue of life stories that offer different perspectives and insights into our lives and ourselves.

But how could a dream experience have such a profound and lasting effect? This question led me to the work of Boris Heifets, associate professor of anesthesiology, perioperative and pain medicine at Stanford University. The dream team is part of Heifets's lab at Stanford, and in addition to investigating anesthesia dreams, he has extensively studied the healing power of psychedelic medicine.

When I met with Heifets, we talked about some parallels between anesthesia dreams and psychedelic medicine, which centres on the role of an experience to change people's thoughts, emotions, and behaviour. People set their intentions and expectations, and have a psychedelic-assisted experience, which may involve enlightenment, emotional pain, or chaos. Then they try to make sense of the profound experience and how to integrate it into their waking lives. Each aspect is an important part of the process and is done with the guidance of a mental health professional. Having an intense, guided experience in this altered state of consciousness can help people who are stuck in endless loops of PTSD, anxiety and depression, and addiction.

With anesthesia-induced dreams, "we've managed to, in my view, create a psychedelic-like experience without the use of a psychedelic," explained Heifets. Comparing these unique dreams to psychedelic medicine, we talk about whether it could be the drug propofol or the dream "trip" that delivers this transformative experience. Is there a biochemical-based or an experience-based explanation? Heifets explained that the anesthetic propofol doesn't have a transformative, mystical effect on its own. "It has to be experiential," he said. It's the personal and often intense dream experience that seems to have this transformative effect. This is important for several reasons. First off, it shows how an experience alone can have significant and lasting effects on our well-being. "If we want to refocus mental health care on experience and transformational change," said Heifets, "we need to be able to demonstrate the importance of that as an isolated concept." Anesthesia-induced dreams do just that.

Next, these unique dreams change how anesthesia is perceived, making use of a technique that's administered every day in ORs around the world. A few extra minutes under anesthesia could reduce post-operative nausea and sedation while providing patients with a safe space to have transformational experiences. "It's no longer anesthesia to facilitate surgery," said Heifets. One way to think about surgery is "controlled trauma," he explained. Something is being removed, added, or replaced. Then there is the experience of surgery "when you close your eyes and put your life in the hands of someone else," he said, "and then you let go."

Heifets explained how anesthesia-induced dreams use this "uniquely pivotal state," when we are vulnerable and malleable, for "post-traumatic growth." It's the flip side of post-traumatic stress. It's the difference between walking away from a pivotal life event like a car crash and thinking, I was saved, versus thinking, I almost died. Anesthesia dreams could be the dose of experiential medicine that has as much promise as psychedelics without its current challenges. However, access to psychedelic-assisted therapy is limited by its high cost.

Exposure Therapy on Fast Forward

HEIFETS AND HIS TEAM discovered that the psychedelic-like experience of anesthesia dreams provides its own kind of dream therapy. For people suffering from PTSD, these dreams seemed to have a therapeutic benefit. To figure out how this worked, I met with Laura Hack, a psychiatrist who uses a number of treatment measures for PTSD. First, I needed to understand the brain activity associated with PTSD and how the condition is typically treated.

PTSD is a stress response to a traumatic event. The event can range from combat trauma or sexual violence to injury or threatened violence. PTSD is characterized by nightmares, flashbacks, and an uncontrollable recurring loop of events that forces a person to reexperience their trauma. Two people can experience the same traumatic event and have completely different reactions to it. One person may walk away relatively unaffected while someone else may develop PTSD. "It's still not entirely clear why that occurs," explained Hack, who is an assistant professor of psychiatry and behavioral sciences at Stanford University. We know that there is some genetic predisposition to PTSD that influences how we react to a traumatic event.

We talked about what happens in the brain when someone has PTSD. During this severe stress response, there is heightened activity in the amygdala, which is part of the fear circuitry in the brain that identifies and regulates how we respond to perceived threats. At the same time, there is decreased activity in the prefrontal cortex, which helps us make decisions and judgements, including whether something is an actual threat that we need to take seriously.

How, then, had anesthesia dreams provided a safe space for people to process their trauma? How was this possible? This required a closer look at frequency 48. When the patients were dialed into this particular state of consciousness, the prefrontal cortex was aroused. Yet at the same time, people under anesthesia were calm and relaxed. Their parasympathetic system was less aroused. In this peaceful state, patients described positive dream experiences. Curiously, this positive experience seemed to happen no matter what their dream was about. It was the experience, not necessarily the dream itself, that was positive.

This gave the dreamers a newfound freedom to process all kinds of memories, which ranged from uncomfortable to upsetting to traumatic, without the usual noise from the external world. Many patients who revisited traumatic memories didn't seem to experience the associated anxiety. So when the traumatic memory was triggered in the brain, it could be relived in a completely new way. This is what the Stanford team discovered in the case series that observed the experiences of Lucas and two other patients suffering from the aftereffects of trauma. The dream experiences of one patient offered some clues as to how anesthesia dreams could be used to treat PTSD.

A few years ago in California, a twenty-six-year-old woman was attacked in her apartment. When the perpetrator approached her with a knife and the woman held up her right hand to protect herself, several tendons in her hand were severed. After the attack, the woman developed acute stress disorder (ASD), which can lead to PTSD. She suffered from recurrent nightmares in which the perpetrator attacked her. There was always the same ending with the woman's hand being stabbed. She slept poorly and suffered during the day. She startled easily, avoided knives, and sobbed inconsolably when she talked about the attack.[3]

Twelve days after the traumatic event, the woman had reconstructive surgery on her hand. In the calm, peaceful state under light anesthesia, she relived the knife attack. She was back in her apartment where her perpetrator had attacked her. She dreamt of showing up at the emergency department, then having surgery to repair the severed tendons. After surgery in the dream, she examined her repaired hand. Then she went home and did some errands with her hand healed. As soon as the dream ended, the woman had the exact dream again. And again. And again. Several times, her dreaming brain hit replay on the traumatic event, which is unlike ordinary dreams, which don't typically repeat something as it was experienced in waking life. Why did the woman's dream keep replaying the traumatic event? One idea has to do with its striking similarities to a common type of therapy for phobias, anxiety, and stress disorders.

A gold standard treatment for PTSD is exposure therapy. Under the supervision of a trained mental health professional, an individual revisits a traumatic event repeatedly over the course of nine to twelve sessions that last about ninety minutes each. Think of it as a desensitization process. It's also called fear extinction. I asked Hack how it works. "There is a new memory that's created," she explained. "It's the same content, but it doesn't trigger the same emotional response." The fear is extinguished from the traumatic memory.

How does the brain achieve this? By changing the brain activity that is associated with PTSD. Prolonged and repeated exposure to a traumatic event increases activity in the prefrontal cortex while decreasing amygdala activity, "increasing your control over the emotional response," said Hack. Through exposure therapy, the traumatic memory is freed from its associated fear.

The same phenomenon seemed to happen during patients' anesthesia-induced dreams. In a relaxed state when there was low arousal, patients revisited traumatic memories without the associated fear and anxiety. It was as if patients created their own internally generated fear extinction process. One thought is that "it's the brain's way of exposing the person to the trauma just like in a prolonged exposure therapy, but in a condensed form," said Hack. Being in a state of low arousal, the patients were able to process their dream content and go through the process of fear extinction.

These calm dream experiences were in stark contrast to post-traumatic nightmares. People with PTSD often experience disturbing dreams in which they revisit a traumatic event when their arousal system is on high. They might panic and bolt awake, trying to escape the situation. "There's no resolution to what happened," said Hack. "It doesn't play any therapeutic role for them." The research group found that with the low arousal of anesthesia dreams, people were given the chance to come to a resolution in a calm and peaceful state. It was like an exposure therapy session that was on fast forward.

While traditional exposure therapy can be effective, it is a long and emotionally painful process with a high dropout rate. Medication is often used to treat PTSD. Yet there are only two FDA-approved drugs typically used for the condition and only 20 percent to 30 percent of users achieve total remission.[4] PTSD is a significant public health issue. In the U.S. alone, 4 percent of men and 8 percent of women will experience PTSD in their lifetime.[5] Could anesthesia dreams be a simple and cost-effective treatment alternative?

While my conversations with the Stanford scientists and physicians focused on their observations in the case series, it was easy to get caught up in the growing excitement over how these profound dream experiences could be used one day to treat a range of mental health conditions, including treatment-resistant PTSD.

After the surgery to repair her hand, the twenty-six-year-old woman felt "wonderful and relaxed." The next night, she had her first normal sleep since the attack, free of nightmares. For the first time, she talked about the attack with her family. On day seven, she had "normal" dreams. Today, she no longer has symptoms of ASD. It's like the fear has been removed from the traumatic memory.

Out of the OR and into the Lab

COULD IT BE THAT instead of simply facilitating surgery, anesthesia could create a safe space for transformative experiences that improve well-being? Over the case series, the team observed the impact of these dreams. "They really change people's beliefs. Symptoms go away," explained Sikka. "It's almost magical. You think this can't be true. I wouldn't believe it if I didn't see it." This made me wonder, could all anesthesia dreams have a therapeutic effect?

Sikka pointed to initial observations of healthy participants in the lab who are having a different kind of impactful experience. Many subjects have contacted Sikka to share that they've changed something in their lives or made a major decision based on their anesthesia dreams. There was usually something weighing on their minds, and they dreamt about it with a "kind of positive reassurance," said Sikka.

Over the past three years, the Stanford team has surveyed almost one thousand five hundred surgical patients and recorded more than nine hundred dream reports. The next step is to study anesthesia dreams out of the OR. In the lab, the team is doing experimental studies to identify biomarkers of this dreamlike state to understand its biological mechanisms. They are adjusting the propofol to pinpoint the EEG frequency associated with these profound dreams. If the experience can be replicated among diverse groups of patients, this brings it one step closer to one day becoming a standardized, scalable therapy. It appears that these transformative dream experiences occur with several other anesthesia.

Heifets told me of another study in his lab that is using psilocybin during anesthesia to drive the process of a transformative experience. Think of dreams like digestion, said Heifets. When we go to sleep at night, our experiences get "digested," flowing out to our cortex. When you have trauma, it's like "something you can't swallow," he said. "You keep choking on this thing and that wakes you up. So you're never fully able to process it." Anesthesia dreams provide a space for this digestion to happen. With psychedelics, people describe a flooding of memories, including unresolved trauma. They use words like purgative and cathartic when they're able to work through difficult memories. Heifets and his team are testing whether the addition of psilocybin to anesthesia pushes content to the surface to be digested while people are in a relaxed, calm state.

For many patients, the traditional therapies don't work. "I see it every day in the clinic, just how much suffering there is from treatment-resistant depression and PTSD. Frustration and feelings of hopelessness," said Hack, who sees patients at the Stanford Translational Precision Mental Health Clinic and the Precision Neuromodulation Clinic within Veterans Affairs, using a variety of measures to guide people to treatment.

In talking to patients like Lucas, I learned how anesthesia dreams quieted people's anxiety and lightened their depression. I discovered how they wiped away symptoms of PTSD, stopping nightmares and cutting the endless loop replaying a traumatic event. It made me wonder, could these dreams have the power to heal?

Chow has started calling anesthesia dreams psychological antibodies. Under anesthesia, while patients are out of touch with the world around them, they are operating in this sphere of internal consciousness. In this calm, relaxed state, the brain attacks the fear that is connected to traumatic or upsetting memories. Maybe a person is dealing with cancer or symptoms of PTSD. Or maybe it's a ballplayer whose injury prevents him from ever pitching again. In these dreams, the person revisits and comes to grips with difficult situations using these psychological antibodies that remove the fear from the memories.

Lucas described anesthesia dreams as wish fulfillment. Zane had always wanted a dog, but their former landlord hadn't allowed pets. Seeing Zane and his brother laughing and playing with Moxie brought Lucas such joy and relief. In 2023, Lucas had another anesthesia-induced dream in the OR. She dreamt that she was a bird soaring above a cove in Maui. The sheltered inlet was superimposed with the cove in California where they had spread Zane's ashes. Lucas had always wanted to bring Zane to Hawaii. She fulfilled her wish in her dream. She remembered the "drum of happy voices" as she watched Zane and his youngest brother playing on the beach. The memory of the dream was just as vivid several years later.

After Zane died, Lucas suffered from anxiety and depression and was diagnosed with PTSD. She had recurrent nightmares in which she tried to save Zane. One time they were at the edge of a cliff. In another dream, they ran down a long corridor as people chased them. Before the nightmare came to its tragic end, she'd wake up screaming. There was never any resolution. Then she had the dream experiences while under anesthesia. A few days after surgery, Lucas felt unbelievably calm. A month later, she no longer fulfilled the criteria for PTSD. Now, several years later, her nightmares have stopped and she is able to process stress in a way she wasn't able to before.

To help me understand this, Lucas described a game that she played as a kid called Don't Spill the Beans. Each player takes a turn placing a bean into a wobbly pot with a careful, steady hand so the pot won't tip and spill the beans. Players go back and forth until the weight of one additional bean upends the whole pot. Lucas's anesthesia dreams prevented things from spilling over. "They give your brain time to process through all those little beans so that you can have a more healthy brain that's lighter," she explained. Lucas believed that this would have given Zane the relief he needed to manage his anxiety and depression a bit better. "I say that they physically cured me of cancer," she said, "but they saved my life with this."

Chapter Ten

THE POWER OF
LITTLE DREAMS

OUR NIGHTS ARE FILLED WITH "LITTLE DREAMS" THAT HAVE their own kind of quiet or subtle revelations. Yet they often go unnoticed, escaping our memory at the shrill sound of our alarm. I learned a few ways to mine these seemingly ordinary dreams to spark creativity, shift perspectives, and gain insights on our lives. I discovered that we have our own dreamer's toolkit filled with easy techniques to make the most out of our dreams, both big and small.

We might choose to chart the course of our lives through personal experiences. My timeline of events includes when I got married, had kids, the carefree summer I camped under the midnight sun near Whitehorse, the years we lived in London, and soon, when I finish this book. So many moments, both big and small, come to mind. Dreams exist on this continuum of experiences, shaping how we see ourselves and where we're going or where we get stuck along the way. Often, dreams express our preoccupations and concerns, illuminating what needs our attention. With our dreaming brain operating in another mode, we think, feel, and experience things differently.[1] I discovered there is a lot to learn from these alternate experiences, and the more we pay attention to our dreams, the more we can get out of them.

While the possible functions of dreams continue to be debated among the great minds in dream research, there are many ways that we can use our dreams. We spend a huge amount of our waking hours mind-wandering and a third of our lives asleep. There are some simple ways to make the most of our rich, full dream lives. Using my own dreams, I tested two popular techniques used for dream analysis: dream journaling and dream sharing.

Over the years, I've been compelled to write down some of my more bizarre or puzzling dreams so I could remember them. My dream journaling, if you could call it that, has been inconsistent, and I've never taken the time to track patterns or elements across my dreams. I'm not very good at keeping a diary, for dreams or everyday life. When I began research for this book, I started to keep better track of my dreams. I was curious to expand my thinking and views. Yet I couldn't help being skeptical. How could the simple act of writing down my dreams influence my waking life? I've had several eureka moments when I've woken up from a dream with a new idea or completely different way of looking at whatever was weighing on my mind. I've also had a few recurrent dreams that reappeared when I least expected it. But what about all of the other forgotten dreams? What nuggets of creativity and candor had I missed?

I kept coming back to something J. Allan Hobson told me during one of our conversations. The late American psychiatrist and pioneering researcher extensively studied the neuroscience of dreaming. When we chatted, he explained the importance of treating subjective experience as data in dream research. It has been more than 125 years since Freud published *The Interpretation of Dreams*, and some might say that dream science still has what Hobson called a "hangover" from contemporary dream research's "understandable skepticism." From our current vantage point in dream science, some of Freud's theories are long outdated and debunked. Yet several of his theories laid the foundation for research that continues to this day. As Hobson told me, there is a chaotic nonsensical aspect to dreams. Yet this shouldn't dismiss their use in scientific study. The neuroscientist recorded his own dreams, amassing more than one hundred volumes.

We have access to our own dream experiences, which can be used as data to study dreams in the lab and at home. We can conduct our own kind of dream experiments to measure different elements and trace memory sources in our dreams. I decided to give it a try. All I needed was paper and a pen and enough discipline to turn my curiosity into a regular habit of journalling.

I imagined a dream journal as an unedited compilation of stories filled with terrifying tales that I'd lived to tell, the exciting adventures that I didn't want to end, and the strange, bizarre happenings that seem to make no sense. While it was interesting to look at individual dreams, I was curious how a series of dreams would highlight parallels between my waking and dreaming lives. Then I could look at different dreams as experiences that progressed the plot of a larger story.

Recently, I had a strange dream that stuck with me for days. I plotted its puzzling details. Then I sat down with a dream researcher to try and make sense of it.

"We bring up what we need"

KELLY BULKELEY IS THOUGHTFUL and soft-spoken with thick eyebrows atop kind eyes and long silvery hair that he ties back. I reached Bulkeley via Zoom at his home outside of Portland, Oregon. He told me how his own dream experiences got him into the study of dreams. As a kid, he had vivid and recurrent dreams. He also had an early interest in science fiction and philosophy, poring over his parents' college philosophy books when he was twelve years old. "There's a lot of things that were nourishing the imagination," he said. In his late teens, Bulkeley noticed a recurring theme of being chased. Whatever situation he found himself in, there was nothing he could do to stop it. In the dream, he thought, "I can't run away. I can't hide," he said. "I can't fight. I can't talk my way out of it."

Bulkeley grew up in the San Francisco Bay Area and during the 1970s and 1980s, dreams were having a moment in the spotlight. There were lots of workshops and books on dreams, and Bulkeley started reading about Freud and Jung's dream theories. As he began learning about his own dreams, "the dreams began changing, and then new things came up, and the chasing diminished," said Bulkley who described a dynamic back-and-forth between waking and dreaming life. "The more I paid attention to my dreams, the more my dreams paid attention to me," he said. "And the dreams became more interesting and changed, and took me in new directions."

In 2009, Bulkeley launched the Sleep and Dream Database (SDDB), a collection of more than forty thousand dream reports that spans the second century to the present. It's a searchable digital library that categorizes dreams in a range of interesting topics. You can compare the frequency of falling dreams by gender, see how political ideology relates to visitation dreams, and customize your own dream analysis.

Work and relationships are common themes that we play out in dreams. "We're trying to juggle a lot of things," said Bulkeley. "Dreams will revolve around those concerns." We can learn a lot by simply paying attention to who shows up the most in our dreams. It's likely that these people are emotionally important to us. This isn't limited to those we're fond of. It's the emotional intensity about the person that matters. It can be positive, negative, or a mix of both. It's also not restricted to those we see frequently. The people we're emotionally attached to might not be in our lives anymore. This is one of the patterns that can reveal what's happening in a person's life, offering some practical value. It's interesting to think how our dreams aren't simply anchored by our physical experiences. Dreams are often more about our ongoing emotional life.

"It does seem like the strongest signal of meaning in our dreams revolves around our relationships," Bulkeley told me. "This is the place where we can see most clearly how dreams accurately reflect meaningful aspects of our waking lives." We talked about how current experiences and challenges are often reflected in our dreams. Beyond these immediate concerns is Jung's idea that our dreams prepare us to be full humans. According to Jung, "Who we are in this current life is a fraction of what we can be and what we potentially are," explained Bulkeley. "Dreaming is the expression of the whole psyche and is ultimately guiding us toward what he called the path of individuation."

When I asked Bulkeley what he thought of Jung's idea, he explained how it feels true to his own experiences. "The weirdest dreams in some ways are the ones that teach you about the magnitude of your psyche," he said. "It's very easy in life to think this is what it is. The way things are right now, the way I am right now. Our dreams are constantly reminding us there's way more than you thought."

I couldn't help but ask one of the questions that has followed me through my research: Why do we dream about past events at certain times in our lives? I'm fascinated by how we take specific memories of our past and stitch them together with recent moments, creating a dreamy tapestry of experience, emotion, and thought. In speaking with sleep and memory researchers, I understood that we might associate a recent memory with something from our distant past, making it fresh in our minds. I wondered if there were other possible reasons. While Bulkeley explained there is no consensus view on the rationale, he shared one idea. "It seems we bring up what we need," he said. "I think it's more of an inductive kind of thing rather than there is this grand master plan."

While time structures our waking lives, Freud believed that the dreaming unconscious works outside the constraints of linear time. In dreams, "The past, the present, and the future, it's all one big swim," said Bulkeley. When we wake up, we benefit from this time bending. "We've had the time to have that bigger perspective on our lives," said Bulkeley. "And I think that prepares us for the day-to-day."

We talked about many motivations for dream journaling. Some of us might be looking for personal insights, while others want to see who keeps showing up in their dreams. At different times, we can feel stuck in different ways. It might be our career or a relationship. "Our dreams do ruminate," said Bulkeley, who has studied dreams, psychoanalysis, and the psychology of religion for decades. He explained how recurrent misfortune dreams are in some ways similar to PTSD nightmares, yet on a much milder scale. One idea is that with PTSD nightmares "there is a chewing it over because it can't be digested," said Bulkeley. "It's a stimulus that can't be cognitively digested. It's just too much." Recurrent misfortune dreams are much milder. They ruminate rather than relive traumatic events. Yet they can still be distressing.

The AI Dream Decoder

BULKELEY IS A RESEARCH advisor for the AI-powered dream journal app called Elsewhere. It has some interesting features including creating sketches of dreams, identifying patterns, and offering insights on recurring dream elements. People can analyze their dreams using Freudian, Jungian, and other interpretation modes to get different perspectives on their dreams. Then Elsewhere generates results based on the principles of each dream analysis model. Elsewhere isn't a substitute for therapy. It's more of a digital education tool for personal growth and self-awareness. I told Bulkeley about the dream I was trying to make sense of, and he talked me through the Freudian and Jungian interpretations generated by Elsewhere.

Freud believed that most dreams are driven by a repressed wish. These wishes can't be fulfilled in our waking lives, so they find their way into our dreams, seeking fulfillment. Freud saw dreams as the "royal road" to a deeper understanding of our unconscious. He believed that dreams reveal our basic instincts, including sexuality, aggression, and narcissism.[2] According to Freud, our dreams aren't supposed to make sense on their own. He concluded that their real meaning could be found in the latent content, the subterranean layer that is hidden below the surface of dreams. According to Freud, the latent content harbours our hidden wishes and instincts.

Jung took an alternate view. According to Jung, our dreams do not disguise their meanings. They reveal what we really think and envision about our own lives. So why, then, are dreams so strange and bizarre? Jung attributed this to our rational mind being out of touch with our psyche. Jungian dream analysis connects us with our unconscious mind using archetypes, images, and metaphors. Freud was Jung's mentor and close friend for many years. Of all things, a disagreement over the nature of dreams contributed to their falling out. As they went their separate ways, so did their dream theories.

I wondered what the different interpretations on Elsewhere would say about my dream. At the time, I was spending most of my waking hours researching and thinking about dreams. I shared one of my particularly bizarre dreams with Bulkeley.

Away

PICTURE IT. MID-FEBRUARY IN the Canadian prairies. I'm driving through a blizzard in a rental car. There is a hole in the floor of the car, and the ice-cold wind nips at my ankles. I'm inching along a two-lane highway that cuts through vast wheat fields. My windshield wipers can't keep up, and the snow accumulates inch by inch until I'm looking at a wall of ice.

Jump cut to a dimly lit bar where my dad once took me. He used to come here during medical school after long nights of studying. There is a dart-board and some neon beer signs and mismatched, wobbly tables. You tell your server how many glasses of beer you'd like by holding up the same number of fingers. It seems there is only one kind of beer to choose from. I hold up two fingers, and my server slams down two tiny juice glasses of beer that splash onto the table. (Clearly, this is a dream, as I'm drinking beer while waiting to pick up my car.) A gunfire of ice pellets hit the bar's frosted windows, and I feel cozy and safe inside, away from the storm.

I have been given a rental car while my own is being fixed. As I sip my beer, waiting for a call from the service department, I pause mid-dream with a sudden realization. I'm dreaming of a rental car because I spent hours online that day, trying to find a car for an upcoming vacation. I know it's all a dream. But I can feel someone staring at me. I have to find out who he is.

I look over at the next table, and there is a man wearing a gas mask. It feels like there are two sides of me operating at once. One side knows who he is while the other side of me needs him to take off his mask. It's a combination of knowing and not knowing. The server comes over, telling me that I have to pay. Now.

I realize that I've lost my wallet, and she tells me to use my credit card that is loaded on my phone. I tap my phone against the machine, and the transaction fails. I'm hit with another realization, and I tell the server that I'm dreaming this because I'm worried about money. She tells me that I still have to pay, huffing as she shifts her weight from one hip to the other while balancing a tray of drinks. From the corner of my eye, I watch the man in the gas mask come closer until he's by my side. Slowly, he reaches for the bottom of his mask. Inch by inch, he begins to reveal himself. I can see his chin now. As he lifts the mask off his face, I bolt awake. I cover my head with a pillow and try to fall back asleep to see who this man is. But he has vanished.

Freud vs. Jung

"THAT'S A VERY COMPLICATED dream," said Bulkeley as I pulled up the results from Elsewhere's different interpretation modes. We talked about four dream elements: driving in the snowstorm, the bar, the server's demand for payment, and the man in the gas mask. Freud and Jung had a lot to say about my dream.

Elsewhere's Freudian interpretation explained that the act of driving, even in a snowstorm, may symbolize my autonomy and control over my journey through life. By dreaming this, I might have wished for "agency and self-direction."[3] The Jungian interpretation saw the rental car as a temporary state, which indicated that I was navigating a transitional point in life and might be searching for clarity on my direction. I assumed that I dreamt of the rental car simply because I'd spent the day looking for one. I found it interesting that I connected the car with the prairies where we used to rent a car and drive for hours, often in snowstorms, to visit family. This included the time that we got a car with a hole in the floor, just like the one in my dream. The car had been the last one on the lot, so we had to take it.

Next, we looked at the bar where my dad once took me. "Of all the places to bring you to hang out for a while," smiled Bulkeley. "I'm thinking about the roadhouse in *Twin Peaks*." That was exactly the vibe. Dimly lit. Cigarette smoke hung in the air. And a Lynchian sinister twist with a man in a gas mask at the next table.

The Freudian analysis imagined a different atmosphere. It focused on the connection with my dad and envisioned the bar as a place of nostalgia and warmth, which could represent a desire for comforting family relationships. "There's this kind of sanctuary from all the mayhem and the snow and the cars," said Bulkeley, adding that the comfortable, familiar bar had a womb-like quality. He explained how Freud disliked anything regressive. So Freud might have said that this was a regressive fantasy. A wish to return to the womb. Maybe I just wanted to have a beer with my dad.

The Jungian analysis agreed with the feeling of nostalgia and family connection. It went on to say that I might have been looking for guidance from my dad in a moment of uncertainty as I drove through a snowstorm in a rental car. I wasn't sure why I had dreamt about this particular bar, but it felt good to be there again.

Next, Bulkeley and I talked about the server who demanded payment even though I had shared my money worries. "There is some real energy there," said Bulkeley, who added that he enjoys these kinds of autonomous dream characters with a lot of attitude. The server showed no sympathy for my money worries. I had to pay. "That's kind of a sassy thing to say," he laughed.

Freud thought of money as a psychological extension of our bodies, explained Bulkeley. Also, Freud would have seen the money as part of the manifest content and looked for its hidden meaning. "The money symbolizes something else," he said. The Jungian interpretation saw this interaction as a symbol of accountability and responsibility. I had to face the practicalities of life like paying for my drinks, even if I understood the nature of my dream. The Jungian analysis highlighted the tension between "awareness and obligation," which might have shown a deeper inner conflict between the "needs of the conscious self with the demands of the unconscious."[4] I was intrigued by the tension between our understanding and our responsibilities in life. I could see how this constant push-pull would find its way into my dream.

I was really curious about the man in the gas mask and wanted to get Bulkeley's take on both interpretations. The Freudian interpretation saw the mask as a symbol of fear or anxiety that I might have around revealing my true self. The Jungian analysis focused on the shadow archetype with the man's hidden identity reflecting parts of my own self that were concealed or unacknowledged. From a Jungian point of view, a mask is an invitation to discover what is behind the mask, explained Bulkeley. This figure seemed like a perfect set up for a Jungian analysis.

Jung saw our persona as a sort of public-facing mask. The front that we put up between our true selves and the social world. My inexplicable feelings of both knowing and not knowing the masked figure is exactly the feeling the shadow evokes, explained Bulkeley. "The shadow is oneself. Just an alienated, neglected, and/or repressed one," he said. For Jung, dreams like this are the awakening, said Bulkley. Jung believed that we learn a lot about ourselves if we connect and listen to these figures.

Bulkeley suggested that this is what I had attempted to do. When I realized it was a dream, I could have tried to leave. But I decided to stay and find out who this person was. "That's a great pivot," he said. As Socrates said, know thyself. Whereas Freud would not have wanted me to try and relate to what I had repressed. He might have decided that my inner moral conscience would be too upset to face the truth about myself if I had seen what was behind the mask. So I woke myself up.

I was curious to see what Bulkeley thought about the cliffhanger of my dream that was cut off by my alarm. "That doesn't feel coincidental," Bulkeley said, shaking his head. He explained how we seem to have a kind of internal clock that knows what time it is. I understood what he was talking about. Every morning, I wake up within minutes of the same time, even on weekends or when I forget to set my alarm. Ending with such a cliffhanger, "that's like the director of the drama knows when to reach the climactic moment," he said. Looking at it through a Freudian lens, it was like a "wish unfulfillment."

Bulkeley stressed that these were only suggestions on how I might look at my dream. Of course, there were many other perspectives that I could take when trying to make sense of my dream story. Ultimately, it is up to the dreamer to decide what resonates with them. That's always the test, he said. I asked him if we are really the interpreter of our dreams. "Ultimately, yes," he said. "I think we're good at it. It's kind of a natural human facility." After all, we are the ones who created them.

While I didn't agree with all of the dream interpretations, they got me thinking in new directions. I was able to revisit forgotten places and moments from my past. And I was surprised and intrigued by the strange dream characters that I had created. Maybe this was the motive that I needed to keep up with my dream journal. It made me wonder, how many of us take the time to record our dreams?

Night Library

I LOOKED AT VARIOUS studies and found that between 14 percent and 24 percent of people have recorded at least one dream in their lives.[5] Less than 5 percent of us record our dreams once a week or more. Some people keep a dream diary more than others. Women remember and record more dreams with a greater interest in dream interpretation than men. When it comes to personality factors, people with a high openness to experience tend to record more of their dreams. In general, people who recall their dreams more often are more likely to keep a regular dream journal.

We might be biased in the dreams we choose to record. It is tempting to focus on the exciting or terrifying ones. It makes me think of the stories I choose to share with friends. There's a tendency to recount stories with an entertaining climax or cliffhanger, causing the most dramatic reactions. It would be pretty dull to tell friends that I spent today sitting at my desk, typing on my laptop, with the big action being the neighbourhood bunny taking a few nibbles of our basil plants. When it comes to our dreams, which stories do we want to remember and share with our waking selves?

There have been several studies on people recording dreams of their ex-partners and deceased loved ones. This includes a remarkable case study of a woman referred to as Barb Sanders by social psychologist G. William Domhoff, who analyzed her extensive series of dreams. The middle-aged woman recorded more than 3,100 dreams over two decades. She had always been interested in dreams and began a journal after her divorce, a difficult time that was punctuated by disturbing dreams.

Domhoff did a content analysis using the Hall/Van de Castle dream coding system, an established dream analysis tool. He conducted interviews with Sanders and several friends, exploring the continuity and discontinuity between Sanders's dreams and her waking life. The case study showed that our dreams often involve people who are important to us, and the way we interact with them in our dream world depends on how we think about them in our waking lives. Sanders's dream series charted the course of her complicated relationships and feelings about men, including anger about the failed relationship with her ex-husband, who died of a heart attack just as she began to forgive him.

Sanders's detailed dream series showed how our dreams express our preoccupations, which are sometimes played out through doom-and-gloom scenarios. Sanders became infatuated with a friend from her playwriting group. When she discovered that he didn't share her feelings, she was devastated. Her dreams reflected her waking hopes, which illustrated how dreams are a continuation of our waking lives. Yet Sanders's romantic dreams of this man did not reflect her waking reality. The case study identified other discontinuities with her waking life. This included her dreams about confidently shooting a gun to defend herself even though she disliked guns and hadn't had much exposure to them. There were dreams of skillfully riding a horse even though Sanders was not a good rider, and growing up, she'd been frightened of the large animals.[6] (Sanders's dream series is available at Dreambank.net along with some interview transcripts.)

The discontinuities in dreams can be sources of creativity. When the dreaming brain puts seemingly random things together, it creates another dimension of possibility and imagination. How does the dreaming brain provide such unique ways of thinking and seeing the world and ourselves? Michael Schredl gave me a simple way of understanding this. In dreams during NREM and REM, "the brain is in a different state, so how you experience subjective things changes," said Schredl, head of research at the sleep laboratory of the Central Institute of Mental Health in Mannheim, Germany. This is another dimension, he explained. If you change your brain physiology, you're also changing how you experience things. This made me think of all the details in my dreams that don't make sense. Instead of dismissing it as nonsense, what if I let my mind pursue these new ideas and lines of thought?

Schredl has been studying dreams for more than thirty years. He is a prolific writer and researcher on the subject, and our interviews spanned many dimensions of dreaming. I was fascinated by the concept of dreams as brainstorming. "You have a lot of ideas, and most of the ideas don't make any sense in your waking life," said Schredl. It's up to our waking consciousness to decide which ideas we can use. I described how the first few minutes of sleep remind me of a dreamy brainstorming session when I'm disconnected from the day's obligations and distractions, freeing my thoughts. But at the same time, I'm still focused enough to recognize and reflect on these thoughts. Schredl said this happens to him during sleep offset when he lies in bed for a few extra moments after he has woken up. Sometimes he gets ideas for papers and articles.

Schredl has chronicled more than eighteen thousand of his dreams, compiling about one hundred dream diaries. He began recording his dreams in 1984 and has used his own lengthy dream series to conduct research as well as gain personal insights. He completed a study on the impact of climate change on dreams and discovered that snow, ice, and hail have decreased in our dreams over the years. In Germany, where he lives, the winters are getting warmer, and this is reflected in dreams. Schredl discovered that most of his pain dreams involve situations that he has never experienced in his waking life. Some themes show up in creative ways, like setting boundaries. He has explored this psychological topic in various dream scenarios. In one dream, his brother came into his room and took something without asking. In another dream, he found himself in a living room with a hole in one of its walls where animals could come and go.

For many months, I recorded my dreams and created my own mini catalogue of dream stories. When I looked at my dreams as a series, I noticed certain themes kept popping up. I dreamt a lot about work, which I learned is quite common. I dreamt about money in various ways. I forgot my bank pin, my credit card bounced, and I overpaid for a puppy of all things. I often paused mid-dream and told myself why I had chosen to dream about a certain topic. This would poke holes in my dream story, and I would realize that it was a figment of my imagination. Yet I never tried to gain control. I always wanted to see where my dream would take me. My dream journal was full of mystery and familiarity, part fact, part fiction, with details from my waking life as well as my imagination.

I thought about how a dream journal can give context to our dreams. It can highlight patterns that might otherwise go unnoticed. This reminded me of when I kept a food diary for a few months to investigate food sensitivites. I hadn't realized what I was consuming and how different foods affected me until I mapped out my daily intake. What ideas, thoughts, or experiences was I trying to process, sometimes again and again, in my dreams? What familiar places did I revisit? What experiences did I recreate in new and unusual ways? If I continued to record my dreams, I could examine them over time and see how my dreams changed along with me. As our relationships, careers, and concerns evolve, so do our dreams.

I discovered the catch. Dream journaling takes work. It requires mental energy in those slumberous moments after waking when all you want to do is hit the snooze button and doze a little while longer. But if you drift off, your dreams might escape your memory and disappear. To make the most of my dream journal, I had to keep up with it, writing down all of the dreams that I remembered, even the dull or uninspiring ones that could be full of surprises when I gave them a closer look. The good news is, the more we record our dreams, the more we tend to recall them. And by remembering and reflecting on our dreams, we're able to use them in our daily lives.

It made me think of how we can use our nightly brainstorming sessions as a business or creative tool. One idea is that the creative process begins with an intense focus on something. Then we pause and allow our intuition, our unconscious, even our dreams to reflect and work on it as well. Bulkeley explained how we practice this back and forth. "There's a rhythm between focus, conscious work, and open-ended unconscious work," he said, adding that if you pay attention to dreams over time, "you can really see that play out in your own life."

In dreams, as in waking life, we might not recognize the obvious. "We're human. We have our blind spots," said Bulkeley. For centuries, cultures around the world have practiced dream sharing to enlighten dreamers and foster connection within communities. It's "applied empathy," said Bulkeley. "It's beautiful. It's hard to describe in the abstract." I had to try dream sharing and see if I could experience the applied empathy that Bulkeley talked about. So I chose another dream from my journal that had been tugging at my attention for weeks. I shared it in my first "dream salon," where some researchers, avid dreamers, and friends helped me figure it out while an artist brought my dream to life.

Little Dreams, Take Two
The Art and Science of Dream Sharing

WITH A LARGE MUG of steaming tea beside my laptop, I settled into the stillness of my house on a Saturday morning, ready to embark on a completely new experience, which caused a flutter of nervous excitement. I'd never shared a dream with a group before. It felt so personal to share my inner thoughts and feelings. Yet I was curious to get other people's views on a dream that I couldn't seem to shake.

Two floors above, my husband and teenage kids were asleep in their rooms. Our silver Labrador dozed in her bed in her usual sleeping position, on her back with her paws in the air, with the occasional twitch or whimper in her sleep. Who knows what wonderful or terrifying dream adventures my family was having as I connected online to join my first dream salon?

I exchanged morning greetings with sleep scientist Mark Blagrove and artist Julia Lockheart who hosted the session from Wales. Blagrove is professor of psychology at Swansea University, while Lockheart is a professor of creative practices at University of Wales Trinity Saint David. Since 2016, they have held dream salons online and in person around the world, including at London's Freud Museum, the Carl Jung Institute in Zurich, and UCLA.

The idea was inspired by the salons in Paris during the surrealist movement in the 1920s. The French poet André Breton encouraged people to celebrate the "omnipotence of dreams" and the unconscious, inspiring freedom of thought and art that veers away from logic and a rationale. Think how we still use the word surreal to characterize what is bizarre and dreamlike. The salons in Paris offered a playful and relaxed space to create, dance, or talk about art over a drink. Blagrove and Lockheart have brought this celebration of free thought and art to the world of dreams.

With DreamsID, which stands for Dreams—Interpreted and Drawn,

Blagrove and Lockheart have put together their own artistic happening that combines art and performance to create an interactive event. I was excited to see how one of their dream salons worked. They went through a rundown of the event. First, I would share a dream with the group. I had a strange one that I'd been saving. Then others would offer their thoughts on the dream. At the same time, Lockheart would paint a picture of the dream, making it visible to everyone but me. I'd have to wait until the end of the session.

Her "canvas" was a double-page spread from Freud's *Interpretation of Dreams*. With permission from the publisher Wordsworth Classics, Lockheart would carefully remove two pages from her thinning copy of the iconic dream book to paint my dream. The book was a sliver of its original size after she had created artwork for about one hundred dream salons. Blagrove would moderate the event while Lockheart did her "visual notetaking" of my dream and the group discussion. We would wrap up with Lockheart explaining her process.

My computer screen became a grid of smiling faces as people logged on from Canada, the United States, and the UK. Joining us were some dream researchers, artists, and avid dreamers who often participated in dream groups. I'd also invited some friends and former classmates from my master's program.

We used the popular Montague Ullman dream appreciation method, which involves several steps that people are encouraged to follow in order. First, a person shares their dream. Then the group can ask any necessary questions so the dream is clear in people's minds. From here, people share their thoughts and feelings if the dream had been their own. They might want to start things off with, "If it were my dream . . ." The dreamer can talk about people's comments or keep their thoughts for their own reflection. Then the dreamer shares what was happening in their waking life around the time of the dream. This includes experiences, concerns, even conversations that might have stayed with them. The group looks for connections between the person's waking and dreaming lives. This could be metaphorical or literal connections. The hope is that the dreamer walks away with new insights on their dream and possibly their life. (If you'd like to give it a try, there are instructions in the toolkit at the back of the book.) To begin the session, I shared my dream with the group.

Release

I'M WEARING A LONG, camel-coloured wool coat, which evokes a feeling of warmth and luxury. It reminds me of a coat that I tried on then left on the rack after I'd seen the price tag. There is a pocket on the bottom inside of the coat that makes me think of a kangaroo's pouch. I'm hiding someone in this large pocket. I have a feeling I know them, and I think it's interesting that I'm hiding this particular person. Yet their identity evades me. I'm so tired from trying to hold on to the details of my dream so I can write about it. I tell myself that I'll remember the person in my coat so I can just enjoy my dream.

The person has been lost for a while, and people are running around me, screaming his name. I recognize panic in people's eyes. Yet I don't say a thing. I burrow my face into my coat, whispering to the person that he's safe with me. I tell myself that I'm doing a good thing rather than something deceitful. My dream-self wakes up to write down my dream, and I relax now that it's recorded for my book.

Suddenly, the beautiful coat and the person hiding inside are gone. I find myself standing in front of a door, staring at a rectangular opening that's like an oversized mail slot. The door leads into a restaurant where I'm trying to get a job. The restaurant owner tells me that I have to fit through the slot if I want to work there or even eat in the restaurant. This is upsetting and unfair. No one can fit through a mail slot. Someone points to a tall, broad-shouldered man who slides easily through the slot. I announce that I don't want to work there. It's a difficult decision when my bank account is empty.

Then I find myself in the middle of nowhere dragging a large sack. I decide to put all of my dreams into the bag, hoist it over my shoulder, and carry them with me into the morning to write about them. The bag keeps getting heavier the more I dream, until I can't walk anymore. Then I find myself near our family place in northern Ontario. I tell myself that it makes sense I'm dreaming this because it's the same walk my family and I took every day during the first COVID-19 lockdown. It's a twelve-kilometre walk with hilly country roads that lead to a golf course. It is early spring and I step onto the crisp, wheat-coloured grass. The brittle branched trees are stripped of their leaves. Yet the warmth of the sunshine on this cold spring day makes it beautiful. Everything feels OK. I see a puddle in the shape of a heart that reminds me of the puddle our daughter found on one of our walks. It's on one side of a rickety wooden bridge overtop a country road. There is no one for miles and I stare at the sun reflecting in the heart-shaped puddle.

I can't walk anymore with my bag overflowing with dreams, so I have to let a few go. I open the bag and watch some dreams seep out like cigarette smoke. In the wispy smoke, I see videos playing of my dreams, but I can't see what they're about. I watch them float through the air before disappearing. Then I wake up.

The "Emotional Temperature" of Dreams

MONTAGUE ULLMAN WAS A well-known psychoanalyst and psychiatrist in New York City who developed the technique to help people work with their dreams. While Ullman believed that dreams are useful in therapy, he also felt that we don't necessarily need an "expert" to help us. We can all become experts on our dreams, and with the help of others, we can open our eyes to different ways of seeing our dreams, gaining different perspectives on ourselves and challenges in life. He believed that we create visual metaphors in our dreams to express our thoughts and emotions. People who aren't personally invested in a dream can help us recognize our dream metaphors.

"The helpful outside emotional support and the stimulation of imaginative input brings the dreamer closer to his own production," wrote Ullman in *Working with Dreams*, which he co-authored with Nan Zimmerman.[7] For many years, Ullman worked in community mental health in the United States as well as Sweden. He ran community dream groups, teaching countless people how to make the most out of their dreams through the collective experience of dream sharing. Dreams offer personal insights by telling us who we are rather than who we think we are, he explained. They provide honest assessments of the "immediate predicament" we find ourselves in at the time of our dream, measuring our "emotional temperature."[8]

After I'd shared my dream, it was time for the group to ask any necessary clarifying questions. Ivana Marzura, a health care software technologist from Toronto, was struck by the constant theme of weight and the burden of carrying my dreams. When she asked if it was heavy to carry someone in my coat, I realized that it was no effort at all. Somehow, the person didn't weigh me down. Health care executive Subo Awan was curious about the person that I was hiding. Awan wondered if it was a child. Or could it be someone I saw in myself? It's like I adjusted my lens and saw that I was hiding a man. Yet the picture in my mind was still blurry and I couldn't figure out who he was.

Lisa Beaudoin, who designs health and wellness solutions, asked if I knew why the person needed my protection or what I was protecting them from. That was hard to say. I'd been so focused on how strange it was to have someone inside my coat that I hadn't considered why they were there. I paused to think about it and had a few sips of my tea. I shook my head. I wished I could answer that.

Tony Discenza, a health administrator and post-secondary educator, asked if it made sense to be wearing such a heavy winter coat. What seemed like a straightforward question had me shift my perspective on my dream. Suddenly, I was aware of everyone running around me in shorts and T-shirts, and I realized that the coat was out of place. So why, then, was I wearing it? I had come to the session with a clear picture of my dream. All of these questions made me realize it was a rough sketch with many missing details that needed to be filled in.

Next, we had people imagine the dream as their own. This brought us back to the theme of weight. Harvard dream researcher Deirdre Barrett pointed out several instances in which weight was prohibitive. I emphasized the large stature of the man who I was concerned wouldn't fit through the mail slot to enter the restaurant. Then in the next scene, I was weighed down by my overflowing bag full of dreams. In both cases, "weight is this potential difficulty in progress," said Barrett, who joined us from Cambridge, Massachusetts. If it was her dream, she would consider the idea of physical as well as metaphorical weight that stopped her from doing something. Barrett found it interesting that the man slid through the opening into the restaurant, and later on, my dreams floated out of the bag like smoke, which evoked a feeling of weightlessness. So in a way, it was a tension between being weighed down while I kept moving forward through the dream.

Margo Perlmutter, an HR executive, explored the theme of weight in relation to life's responsibilities like family and finances. She talked about the constant balancing act of making decisions with the best interests of your family while staying true to yourself. "I would feel the pressure of not compromising myself," she said, "along with the weight of being a mom and taking care of my kids." I had been so wrapped up in the strange events of my dream that I hadn't considered any themes that ran through it. I was curious and at the same time confused about the theme of weight. Did it represent something that weighed on my mind?

Marzura thought about obligation in relation to protecting the person in my coat and being torn about a job that didn't align with my values as I stared at my empty bank account. There was also my obligation to remember and record my dreams for this book, which I weaved into my dream story. Then I was released from this heaviness of responsibility as I walked alone on the barren golf course. When I saw the sunshine reflected in the heart-shaped puddle, I was somehow released from these burdens. If it had been Marzura's dream, she would have noticed the moments where she forgot about work, let go, and just enjoyed herself.

Next, we talked about the long winter coat. It reminded Barrett of a heavy swing coat that her mother wore when Barrett was a child. When she was about five years old, Barrett would stand underneath the coat, thinking she was completely hidden, unaware of her legs that stuck out. Her grandmother had a camel-coloured coat, and Barrett would snuggle up to her. In both cases, a maternal figure gave a feeling of comfort. "If it were my dream, I'd notice that I'm now the one wearing the coat and sheltering people under it," said Barrett. I'd forgotten that my mom had a similar long coat when I was a kid. I used to think it was so glamorous. I loved trying it on and walking through the house as the coat dragged behind me.

Discenza reminded us how inappropriate the clothing was, which would have caught his attention had it been his dream. In dreams, Discenza often has "on stage in my underwear moments," he said. If he found himself in a heavy coat, he would panic over what he was wearing underneath in case he had to take it off. Discenza told me about his vivid and recurrent dreams, which sometimes bring him closer to people that he has lost. He described visits from his grandparents in his dreams, which evoked a feeling of connection, even if it was accompanied by a pang of grief.

Blagrove paused from moderating the conversation and pointed out that Freud would have liked my fulfilled wish of getting a coat that I'd wanted in waking life. I had really wanted that coat. So much so that I had taken it off quickly after I'd seen the price tag. I hadn't wanted to get too comfortable in it.

Deirdre Daly joined us from London, England. She was interested in the mix of emotions at different points in my dream. Daly said she would feel a real intimacy toward the person she was hiding in the coat. "I'm rescuing them, and I would feel real love and joy at this strong bond between us," said the lecturer in academic literacies at Goldsmiths, University of London. It was interesting how an innocuous object like a coat could prompt such different reactions within us.

This comfort and warmth was in stark contrast to the anxiousness that Daly felt in the next scene of my dream when the restaurant owner insisted anyone could fit through the mail slot. "I'd feel sad that I couldn't be [me]," she said. The third scene gave her a mixed feeling of loss and happiness. "A little sense of loss, of letting go of something, but also a real sense of enjoying the memory of something," she said. If it was her dream, she would think about the idea that "the things that are gone from my life, I still have them as memories."

Paul Stocks, senior lecturer at Goldsmiths, University of London, was struck by the mail slot as a metaphor for a job interview. For him, it brought up the idea of having to fit into a work culture in order to get a job. He offered the example of feeling the pressure at work to fit in, from the need to talk about football results on a Monday morning to drinking pints in the pub on Friday after work. For me, it was more of an ontological what-does-it-all-mean kind of thing. It was a tension between the financial obligations of everyday life and finding work that had meaning. "I'm going to think of that metaphor every time I go for an interview for the rest of my life," said Stocks with a smile.

For the next step in the process, I shared what was happening in my life around the time of the dream. Our son had applied to university, while our daughter had just started high school. I had been spending a lot of time thinking and writing about dreams for this book. At the same time, I was exploring new work opportunities. I paused and thought about Barrett's question: Was there anyone in my life who needed protection? The answer was obvious. Yet I hadn't put it together in my mind. My husband was awaiting the results of his annual echocardiogram. He's fine now, but several years ago he had emergency heart surgery to remove a benign tumour. This was followed by a long recovery and all the worry and turmoil that went with it.

Maybe in my dream, I was acting out how I could protect him, said Barrett. I zoomed in on the dream image of the person inside my coat. Could it be Dimitri? I shook my head at the thought of the heart-shaped puddle. I'd assumed it was just a snapshot of the puddle our daughter found on one of our long walks during the COVID-19 pandemic. I often do this. Connect dreams with moments in my waking life. Usually, it offers enough of an explanation to satisfy my curiosity.

We returned to the winter coat. Awan pointed out how I was protecting the person in my coat while the chaotic scene played out around me. Could it represent self-confidence, asked Awan, who said she is fascinated by dreams, even though she rarely remembers her own. I paused for a moment to consider this. I'd been so wrapped up in what I was doing in my dream that I hadn't thought about what I was feeling. While I wouldn't have seen myself as self-confident, I'd had a gut feeling that everything would be OK. I guess deep down, I'd known that I could deal with the chaos around me.

"You've got this shield, and that can protect you and the person with you," she said. "In order to protect someone, you have to have confidence in yourself to do it, and you have to take the risk to do it, and I think that takes a lot of guts." I hadn't thought about it like that. Everyone in my dream was in a state of panic and it was quite shocking that my bank account was empty. When the heart-shaped puddle reflected the sunshine, I realized that despite everything, life was good.

Perlmutter thought it was interesting that I released some of my dreams where I used to walk with my family. She pointed out how I had been working on my book a lot, which meant less time to spend with my family. "It's like the bag of dreams is the weight of this book," said Perlmutter. When I was back on the walking path, I was able to release some of the dreams that had been weighing me down.

The group took a look at the last scene when I watched the videos of my dreams float through the air before they disappeared. I'd been unable to see what the videos were about. Barrett pointed out my intermittent awareness throughout my dream. Yet I hadn't tried to gain control. Often in my dreams, I tell myself or other dream characters why I'm dreaming something as it plays out. At some point, my excitement to see what happens next takes over, and I continue on with my dream. Barrett encouraged me to try and build on this semi-lucid perspective. Then I could work at guiding my dreams and make new discoveries. I'm going to give it a try. I had really wanted to see those dream videos before they floated away.

Canvas of Dreams

ALMOST TWO HOURS AFTER the salon began, Lockheart put down her brush. She had finished painting my dream, and was ready to take us through her creative process. (If you'd like to follow along, you can see Lockheart's painting in a blog post on my website, karenvankampen.com.) Lockheart had chosen the two-page canvas from her well-loved copy of Freud's *The Interpretation of Dreams* based on the shape of the blocks of text. Some pages had diagrams or footnotes while others had headings or solid blocks of text.

For my dream, Lockheart chose one page with solid text and the opposite page with three sections to reflect the montage of events. She pointed to the page with solid text. There I was in the voluminous coat from my dream. A face peered out from the coat. In their hair, she had circled Freud's words "I conceal a person," which eerily reflected the scene. Inside the coat, she had circled "distract attention." The words came from sentences that were stacked on top of each other, which made it all the more surreal. A flurry of wide-mouthed faces surrounded me, and I felt the energy of their panic and screams.

She pointed to another image of me, on the opposite page, with my hair blowing in the wind. My dreams floated out of an open bag that was on my back, caught up in the gust of wind. At the top of the bag were Freud's words "in my own inner self" circled in black. Lockheart used the break between paragraphs to create the mail slot, which also acted as a door. This let us look into the restaurant at the man who had slipped through the opening. He sat among other patrons enjoying their food.

The next block of text featured the golf course, a big blue sky filled with fluffy clouds, and the path that I followed in my dream. There was a hole as part of the course, and it circled the words "final cure of a solution," which Lockheart had sketched before I mentioned Dimitri's heart surgery. This elicited a few smiles and headshakes from the group as we scanned Freud's words that somehow reflected my dream story. Another strange coincidence was the heart-shaped puddle that Lockheart painted in red rather than blue. "It's almost like there is a kind of communication from Freud coming up over the centuries," she said. Blagrove felt that Jungians would enjoy the synchronicity of Freud's words incorporated into the painting.

Freud, on the other hand, might have pushed me to interpret not only the content but the mechanism of my dream, suggested Blagrove. While I had fulfilled my wish of getting the luxurious winter coat, I kept reflecting on waking life during my dream. "Freud would say you're not actually in the moment," said Blagrove. My attention was divided between my waking and dreaming worlds. I reflected on past experiences while I remained aware of my obligation to remember my dreams to write about them. Dreaming was work rather than escape. It was the opposite of mindfulness, explained Blagrove. In life, "we all have unquiet minds," he said. We daydream about the past and the future, which pulls us away from the present. In my dream, my mind was cluttered with the same kind of busyness and distraction.

The camera panned across Lockheart's canvas. My long winter coat anchored the page while the wide-mouthed faces and soft, swirling lines created energy and movement. My tight-lipped straight face revealed nothing of my secret and the man I hid in my coat. Lockheart had brought my dream to life. Yet the painting captured so much more than my original dream. I never would have considered the weight and burden that I carried. I was so focused on connecting details to my waking life that I hadn't realized their possible significance.

Maybe I was hiding my husband, trying to keep him safe as we awaited the results of his echocardiogram. Maybe the mail slot showed that I wasn't willing to compromise, that I needed to wait for meaningful work. (The empty bank account was still worrisome, though.) At the end of the session, I was left with this gut feeling that everything would be fine, even if there were many more mail slots I had to try and fit through, so to speak. Until talking about the dream, I hadn't considered the feelings it evoked. "The painting is the collective moment," said Lockheart. It's like I started with a rough mental sketch of my dream, and with everyone's comments and questions, encouraging me to see things differently, it had come alive in technicolor.

Found Objects

A FEW DAYS LATER, I reached Blagrove at his home in Wales. Now that I had experienced dream sharing, I wanted to learn how it fit into the scientific study of dreams. Blagrove's own dream research could be traced back to his student days at Cambridge University. He was about to graduate from natural science and psychology when a friend gave him *The Innocence of Dreams* by psychoanalyst Charles Rycroft. In the book, Rycroft argued that dreams innocently tell us about our lives.

"The dream just tells you like it is in a metaphorical way," said Blagrove, "and I was so fascinated by that." At the time, Blagrove was immersed in biology and psychology. His friend, a theology student, shared a different way of thinking. Blagrove even went to a Freud analyst to talk about his dreams. Then for his PhD, he investigated the meaning of dreams and their association with waking thought, emphasizing that dreams can in fact be meaningful even if they don't have a function.

Blagrove's first experience with dream sharing happened by chance. In 2008, during the International Association for the Study of Dreams conference, he attended a dream group where he shared one of his dreams. Blagrove had dreamt that he was given some CDs by his wife. On the cover was a classic image of the Dutch master painter Rembrandt in his heavy gown and oversized hat. Someone in the group asked Blagrove what the hat could possibly mean to him. Blagrove had just been promoted to professor and was about to become department chair at Swansea University. Suddenly, he lined up the image of Rembrandt with himself in an academic cloak and ceremonial hat. Then someone else asked if Rembrandt might be associated with REM sleep. "That just floored me," he said with a smile.

When I began to research studies on dream sharing, I discovered that it is quite common to talk about your dreams with others. One study by Michael Schredl found that about 27 percent of subjects shared their dreams frequently.[9] This made me wonder, why are we compelled to talk about our dreams with others? Could dream sharing serve a purpose?

I needed to look at the experience of sharing a dream as well as reflecting on someone else's dream. For the dreamer, there are two types of aha experiences, said Blagrove. First, you have a sudden realization of where a certain image comes from, like Rembrandt's hat that Blagrove associated with his new academic appointment. The second aha experience is when the dream reveals something about yourself, like the physical and metaphorical weight that I carried in my dream.

Dreams don't simply replay what we already know, explained Blagrove. "Dreams are based on your concerns and emotions, and they produce something novel," he said, which makes them so striking and important if we take the time to consider them. Our dream metaphors can help us make sense of waking life.

Blagrove sees dreams as "magical, original screenplays." Yet they're not like the plot line of just any movie. It's like a film that was made just for you. It's linked to your life, portraying your emotions and concerns in a metaphorical way. In dreams, "we produce these stories without any artifice," Blagrove said. When we're awake, we create stories deliberately. Yet in dreams, there is no deliberation, he explained. What makes dreams so special is that they give context to our lives by exploring thoughts, feelings, and experiences in different ways. Through dream sharing, we shine a spotlight on these metaphors that seem to be telling us so much.

In 2016, Lockheart devised her own visual note taking for their sessions, "returning the dream to a visual form," said Blagrove. In the process, Lockheart discovered what the surrealists called objets trouvés, found objects within her works of art. These came in the form of "found" language from Freud that often reflected people's dreams. Lockheart had imagined that she would find words related to dreaming in Freud's iconic dream book. But she quickly realized that the connections were much more unusual and relevant to a particular dream. "I was making found poetry from the text while also drawing images," she told me during one of our chats. Then came an unexpected discovery that had Lockheart and Blagrove question the purpose of dreaming.

I Feel for You

THE INITIAL GOAL OF the dream salon was to offer insights to the dreamer, who was given a painting of their dream to take home and continue to reflect on. He and Lockheart thought of it as a "social service for people to help them understand their dreams," said Blagrove. At the time, research was focused on the effect of dream sharing on the dreamer. One study found that sharing a dream heightened intimacy and trust within a relationship if the other person's reactions were supportive and free of judgement.[10] Another study found that people shared dreams mostly with romantic partners, friends, and family, which could enhance intimacy in a relationship or provide some stress relief.[11]

There are many reasons to share our dreams. Maybe we are looking for some immediate relief from a nightmare by retelling it. Or maybe it's the bizarreness of a dream that compels us to talk about it. One study found that people shared dreams to entertain, to uncover the meaning of a dream, or to let someone know what was on their mind.[12] Sharing something as personal as a dream can build connection and empathy. Seeing a dream through someone else's eyes can shift people's perspectives on their dreams and possibly on themselves. But what about the person who listens to the dream? Does the act of sharing a dream have an effect on them?

A recent study discovered the most common reaction to someone else's dream was laughter or amusement, at 35 percent of respondents. This was followed by sympathy at 23 percent. Subjects rarely reported negative reactions. Interestingly, only 9 percent of reactions were neutral or described as no reaction at all. Then the researchers examined the emotions that people experienced when listening to someone's dream. Astonishment was the most common emotion at approximately 83 percent. About 63 percent of the study's subjects described a feeling of joy when they heard someone's dream. They also reported feelings of anxiety and grief quite frequently.[13] This made sense to me, as I thought about how deeply personal a dream can be, and how sharing this might create a moment of closeness and affinity.

Blagrove told me about a deeply moving dream that a woman shared in one of the early dream salons. The woman found herself walking along a street in the evening. She followed a row of streetlights until she came to a red door. The woman's daughter and boyfriend stood beside her. It was their new home. Her daughter walked through the door with her boyfriend while the woman stood outside by herself and thought, Where is my home?[14]

Blagrove and Lockheart were overcome with empathy for the woman. "We just felt so much for her," said Blagrove. The experience brought him back to the fundamental question of why we dream. This got us talking about the incredibly complex films that we produce while we are asleep. Why do we work so hard to create these detailed dream productions? Why not stick with a simple storyline?

In the ongoing study of why we dream, scientists continue to look at the within-sleep and the post-sleep effects of dreaming, which generate so many questions to explore. Do we consolidate memories, process emotions, or prepare for potential risks while we sleep? Then do dreams serve their purpose even if we don't remember them? Or could they also serve a purpose if we recall them after we've woken up? Is a possible function also a possible use? Are dreams designed so we can use them in our lives, specifically to share them with others? Whether dreams are accidental, interesting by-products of sleep or personal stories written with the help of our "emotional" brain, do they serve a purpose when we tell them?

The Evolution of Dream Sharing

BLAGROVE POINTED TO THE evolution of storytelling. What began as rudimentary stories more than a hundred thousand years ago have developed into these incredibly complex narratives, said Blagrove. Storytelling progressed along with language, becoming more intricate and imaginative. It moved beyond simple tales of everyday life to the wild realms of fiction, building excitement and suspense in audiences who couldn't predict where stories would take them.

Maybe dreams have had a similar kind of evolution, said Blagrove. Dreams may have started as mimetic, he suggested, copying the waking world as early stories might have done. Maybe early humans had quite simple dreams, putting together a few basic images and possibly acting out what they did during the day. Then once dreams became more complicated works of fiction, they aroused the same kind of suspense and intrigue as storytelling. If this evolution is possible with our waking stories, why not our dream stories? Dreams evolve over a person's lifetime. In childhood, dreams are quite simple. Yet they develop along with us, building complex, changing narratives with casts of diverse characters exploring difficult themes and emotions.

So what could be the evolutionary benefit to sharing dreams? Keeping with the analogy of storytelling, maybe dream sharing is like other forms of artistic expression that let us bond with others. This connection might attract us to another person, serving as a type of sexual selection, suggested Blagrove. Studies have found that storytelling and artistic virtuosity are features that attract some people to others.[15] Dream sharing might work in a similar way.

It made me wonder, how do we bond over a dream? We talked about the concept of dreams as a kind of fiction that people can explore and experience together. It made me think of how I bond with friends over favourite movies and books. My husband often says quotes from our favourite movies, which remind us of the films as well as watching them together.

I learned that dream sharing is its own collective experience. Yet dreams aren't like other pieces of fiction. They can be deeply personal. If someone chooses to share their dream with us, it might increase our understanding and empathy for their vulnerabilities and situation in life.[16] What if the point of producing these nightly stories is to share them so we can find new metaphors to understand waking life? What if the effect could be just as powerful for others?

Blagrove and Lockheart investigated the relationship between dream sharing and empathy. In 2019, Blagrove and Lockheart conducted two studies to test this connection using the Ullman dream appreciation method. First, they looked at empathy as a personality trait. They found that trait empathy is significantly associated with how much people share their dreams, listen to other people's dreams, and their attitude toward dreams. Then they looked at state empathy, which is the level of empathy that we feel toward another person at a certain time. They looked at the state empathy of the dreamer as well as people reflecting on another person's dream. They discovered a significant increase in people's state empathy when they discussed other people's dreams. Dream sharing gives us a boost of empathy for others.

In dreams, we write stories that are part fiction, part non-fiction, a mix of the strange and bizarre with the very real emotions and concerns from our everyday lives. Maybe dreams are like literary works that have been found to increase empathy in readers as they invest in the story and the lives of its characters.[17] Maybe a purpose of dreams is to share and experience them together.

The last leg of my journey through dreamland ventured into the next frontier in dreaming: dream engineering. We spend our days guiding our minds to learn, create, and heal. Dream engineers make this possible in our sleep.

Chapter Eleven

DREAM ODYSSEY

IN JANUARY 2019, A SLEEPING UNDERGRADUATE STUDENT FROM Northwestern University sent an important message from the dream world, opening the lines of communication to this remote inner realm that is guarded by sleep.

It was almost 9 a.m. when Christopher Mazurek, the nineteen-year-old undergrad, returned to Ken Paller's Cognitive Neuroscience Laboratory for yet another nap. Mazurek was part of a study to test whether it was possible to communicate with a dreamer. This required instant feedback from subjects rather than retrospective dream reports. To attempt this ambitious feat, Paller had designed the study using the rare and magical phenomenon of lucid dreaming.

In a lucid dream, you gain awareness of your dream state. You're hit with the lightning-bolt realization that everything around you is a dream. There are varying degrees of lucidity that range from awareness to control. In a full-blown lucid dream, you are fully cognizant, explained cognitive neuroscientist Benjamin Baird. You have some of your waking faculties at your disposal. A triad of cognitive abilities come together when you are in a complete state of lucidity. First off, there is the awareness that you are in a dream. Then there is the sense that you have control of your attention as well as your actions. Certain complex thought processes are at your disposal, letting you make decisions and reflect on past feelings and events. Your episodic memory lets you recall past waking and dreaming experiences. Think of it as regaining memory of who you are. This is why lucid dreamers can remember that they are sleeping in a lab, hooked up to electrodes, and know the mission they intend to carry out in their dreams.[1]

Most lucid dreams occur during REM sleep while the body is paralyzed and the eyes dart back and forth behind closed lids. The groundbreaking lucid dreaming studies in the mid-1970s by Stephen LaBerge and Keith Hearne showed that lucid dreamers can use eye signals to message the waking world and indicate they are lucid. But can people use eye signals to communicate between the waking and dreaming worlds? Is it possible for lucid dreamers to hear a question, process what they're being asked, and give an answer by moving their eyes during REM while remaining in a dream state? Paller and his team were determined to find out. They compared their experimental goal to trying to talk to an astronaut who is in another world, a place that is fabricated from memories in the brain.[2]

Mazurek was among the dream voyagers of the study. When we met, he told me about his longtime fascination with lucid dreaming. He had been trying to lucid dream since high school, trying all sorts of techniques. During the day, he would do reality checks, staring at his hands, which often appeared with the wrong number of fingers during a dream. Mazurek would wake himself up in the middle of the night, then fall back asleep, focused on having a lucid dream. None of his techniques seemed to work.

Then he joined Paller's lab as a research assistant and signed up to be a subject in the lucid dreaming study. Around the same time, Mazurek started a dream journal. Every morning for five years, he recorded his dreams, filling several notebooks with detailed accounts. Mazurek found that journaling helped him remember and reflect on his dreams, which is thought to help people become lucid. By distinguishing between our waking and dreaming experiences, we are more likely to notice when we are in a dream. Also, journaling highlighted certain patterns that helped with lucidity. Mazurek noticed many dream reports about his childhood home, which became a trigger for awareness in his dreams. If he dreamt of being in his old house, he would pause and think, I'm supposed to be in my dorm room or the lab, which would signal that he was dreaming.

Border Crossing

BY THE TIME MAZUREK walked into the lab that January morning for another nap, he was getting good at navigating and guiding his dreams. Cognitive neuroscientist Karen Konkoly lived about a twenty-five-minute walk from the university. It was a cold, dark walk that morning, and she came into the lab with a large coffee and green smoothie, ready to observe another one of Mazurek's naps. Around 8:30 a.m., Mazurek arrived. By this point, Konkoly had monitored more than a dozen of Mazurek's naps, waiting for his rapid-fire eye movements to signal lucidity before she attempted to communicate with him as he traversed through the dream world.

As one of the first authors of the study, Konkoly had spent countless hours staring at EEG readouts of sleeping subjects, waiting for that moment to communicate with another dimension. "The sensory connection and disconnection between these two worlds is so fascinating," said Konkoly, whose excitement about the science of dreaming is infectious. We had several Zoom calls while she was living for about a year on the Big Island of Hawaii. She spoke rapid fire with quick hand gestures, sharing her extensive knowledge and imparting her fascination with the mysterious and often confounding dream state. "You can pass information from one dimension to another—from one world to another—and it can appear in completely idiosyncratic ways," she said.

Imagine a car alarm goes off somewhere on your street while you sleep. Maybe you decide that the sound is unimportant, and as you keep sleeping, you incorporate the sound into your dream. While it may be the same monotonous beeping as a car alarm that goes off on my street in the middle of the night, I might choose to integrate the sound into my dream as the high-pitched squeal from a novice saxophonist while you might transform the same sound into an ambulance siren. "It's a true signal from another place," said Konkoly. "The way that it manifests in your dream just has to do with you."

Konkoly was always fascinated by dimensions of consciousness and reality. She grew up outside of Philadelphia and became interested in dreams when she was in high school. Konkoly won an essay contest that awarded her a Barnes & Noble gift card. She used it to buy a book on lucid dreaming and learned how to become lucid.

Now when she gains awareness in her dreams, Konkoly searches for a dream guide to ask existential questions. One time, she asked a dream guide if she could meet her higher self. In the dream, there was a towering tree with a door. Konkoly peeled away the layers of the tree door and found a coffin. She pried open the coffin door and came face-to-face with her deceased self. She asked her deceased self what she wished she had known earlier in life. Konkoly discovered that she wished she had listened more.

In another lucid dream, Konkoly asked to see her subconscious. She appeared in the lobby of an office building in New York City. Instead of the quintessential lobby plants, she found plastic mannequin heads in planters. She decided that the situation was a farce. Konkoly couldn't believe that this was her subconscious. Then she spotted an elevator. After fighting to stay awake in the elevator, she descended to the bottom floor. The doors opened onto a massive deep-purple amphitheater. Along the floor were triangles, each with an eye staring back at her. Then a voice bellowed, "You are inside a neuron star." She had reached her subconscious. These days, Konkoly has about one lucid dream a month. She spends a lot of her time studying the dreams of subjects like Mazurek.

As a research assistant in Ken Paller's lab at Northwestern, Mazurek was familiar with the set-up and experimental protocol. Konkoly stretched a blue mesh cap over his head. It had thirty-two built-in electrodes to pick up brain waves during different sleep stages. This eliminated the need to measure and place electrodes individually. Mazurek went into a tiny bedroom that was fashioned out of a Faraday cage. Originally, it had been built for wake studies that could be compromised by electromagnetic interference. Its white metal corrugated walls were soundproof, which came in handy for sleep studies. Mazurek lay down on the futon. On her way out, Konkoly turned off the lights. The metal door was so heavy that she had to shove it closed with her hip. She sat down at her computer, spoke to Mazurek through a baby monitor, and began the usual pre-sleep lucid protocol.

Mazurek was trained on the Targeted Lucidity Reactivation (TLR) procedure, which uses sound cues to encourage lucidity. TLR is part of the growing field of dream engineering, which uses technology to help us change our dreams. Before falling asleep, subjects like Mazurek listened to recorded prompts of Konkoly's quiet, calm voice, asking them to be critically aware of their surroundings and experience. The prompts were played along with a series of high-pitched ascending beeps. Then these sounds were replayed when the EEG readout indicated a subject was in REM sleep.

TLR is similar to Targeted Memory Reactivation (TMR), which uses sensory stimulation to reactivate a recent memory during sleep. The mind has a tendency to wander during the day, drifting from one thought to another. It's thought that the same thing happens during sleep. TMR uses stimuli such as sound or light to focus the dreaming brain on a particular memory.

TLR uses the same principles. A memory is linked with a sound, and when the sound is replayed, it triggers the memory. For this study, the cued memory was a reminder for subjects to be critically aware of the world around them. When they heard the sound during REM sleep, the hope was that subjects would become aware of their dream state. "The point is to enter a lucid mindset," said Mazurek. "Start paying attention to what's going on around you, and if it's strange, you might be in a dream." As part of the pre-sleep training, Mazurek and other subjects practiced answering math questions using eye movements. During naps, questions would be chosen randomly so subjects couldn't anticipate the answers.

Sitting in front of her computer on the other side of the corrugated metal wall, Konkoly began the TLR procedure. Mazurek lay in the dark with his eyes closed as three beeps increasing in pitch were played through the computer at the end of the futon. Then a recording of Konkoly's calm, quiet voice instructed, "As you notice the signal, you become lucid. Bring your attention to your thoughts and notice where your mind has wandered. . . . [pause] Now observe your body, sensations, and feelings. . . .[pause] Observe your breathing. . . . [pause] Remain lucid, critically aware, and notice how aspects of this experience are in any way different from your normal waking experience."[3]

The beeps along with the recording were repeated four times. Then about every minute, only the beeps were played. This happened several times.

Konkoly watched Mazurek's EEG readout as he drifted into Stage 1 sleep. His breathing deepened. His eye movements slowed down. As a subject, he was an amazing napper who fell asleep quickly in the lab. Konkoly observed Mazurek in Stage 2 for about twenty minutes. He bounced back and forth between Stage 1 and 2 and woke up a few times.

Ground Control, Do You Copy?

JUST OVER AN HOUR later, Mazurek entered REM sleep, the fourth and final sleep stage, when lucid dreaming usually occurs. Konkoly played the auditory cue twice—the three ascending beeps along with the recording of her voice that encouraged Mazurek to be critically aware of his surroundings. Mazurek had a micro-arousal, which is a brief awakening during sleep, and Konkoly stopped signaling. Then he fell back asleep quickly. Usually, Konkoly would wait until a subject had another set of rapid REM eye movements to get the protocol going again. With Mazurek, there was no need to wait. As soon as he drifted off, he messaged with staccato left-right eye movements. Mazurek repeated the trained series of eye movements six times, an explicit signal that he was lucid.

I asked Konkoly to describe the experience of receiving a message from the dream world. She told me how she often stared at an EEG readout for hours, waiting for that magical moment. "They're in another world, and I'm over here," she said. Then suddenly, there was the signal she had been waiting for, shot through the darkness. "And they're talking to me, even though they're in a completely other universe." She found the lucid dreaming study suspenseful compared to a typical sleep study where participants could only share their dream experiences once they had awakened. To make things even more exciting, Konkoly had been in grad school for only four months.

The grad student discovered that it was a challenge to identify the EEG patterns associated with a lucid dream. Sleep is scored by reviewing EEG activity in thirty-second intervals. When she tried to pinpoint a lucid dream, it was like sleep staging on the fly. Everything was happening so fast. When she observed a sleeping subject, Konkoly had to decide if they were sending the practiced signal for lucidity. Or was she observing the naturally occurring rapid eye movements during REM? Or maybe the person was awake, which generated an EEG readout that was remarkably similar to REM sleep. Seeing only thirty seconds of activity at once on a computer screen required a split-second decision whether a message was being sent from the dream world. With Mazurek, his eye signals were extremely clear, and Konkoly was certain that he was sending her a message.

With his body asleep on the other side of the metal wall and his mind exploring the dream world, Mazurek found himself inside his favourite video game, *The Legend of Zelda*. As he walked through a canyon, he heard a disembodied voice. It was the recording of Konkoly's calm voice, and it emanated from the environment of the simulated game. For other subjects, a different recording played through a car radio or was described as the voice of God or the narrator of a movie.

In the video game, Mazurek suspected that it was a dream. Then he was overcome by a strange sensation. "I lost control of all my muscles," he explained. "There was a roaring sound of blood rushing to my ears."[4] Mazurek's vision darkened as he heard a math problem: eight minus six. As Mazurek focused on the problem, he lost sight of what was happening around him. He flicked his eyes back and forth—left-right, left-right—for an answer of two. A computer algorithm chose another math problem randomly, which happened to be eight minus six. Again, Mazurek's rapid eye movements darted left-right, left-right to signal an answer of two.

Konkoly's voice had found Mazurek in his dream. He had processed the math questions and messaged the correct answers back to her. Konkoly's first reaction was sheer excitement. The math problem only allowed for one correct answer. Could it really be possible? Had they actually messaged back and forth between the dimly lit lab and Mazurek's dream? She would have to wait for the report from independent sleep scorers to find out.

Late one night, Paller asked Konkoly to put together a slide deck of the study's results. Then a couple of days later, Konkoly walked into the undergraduate class where she was a teaching assistant for Paller. The professor was showing the students Konkoly's PowerPoint of the eight minus six math problem. The results were in. Mazurek had answered Konkoly from his dream. That cold January morning in Evanston, Illinois, a newly minted graduate student and an undergraduate subject had opened the lines of communication between the waking and dreaming worlds.

When Mazurek shared the experience with me, he described it as a totally different realm of existence. "As different as space is from life on earth, as dreams are from reality. But the thread of consciousness still connects them," said Mazurek. During the experiment, it was like having a foot in both worlds at once, he said. "Being within a dream but knowing there's a world out there, there's someone actively talking to me and I'm talking back by moving my eyes." He shook his head and smiled. "There's not many other experiences like that I can think of."

Paller discovered their experiment was not the only one of its kind. At the same time, three other groups of researchers were using different types of complex questions and communication strategies to interact with lucid dreamers. This began an international collaboration, with the American team joining forces with groups in Germany, the Netherlands, and France. Across the four studies, there were thirty-six participants, which included novice and experienced lucid dreamers.

The German team recruited ten experienced lucid dreamers with at least once lucid dream per week. Before they were run in the lab, subjects completed Morse code training over the internet. They learned how to decode numbers zero to nine, "P" and "M" for plus and minus, and practiced answering math problems using eye movements. In the lab, the German team transmitted math problems using Morse code, tapping out the messages with flashing red and green LED lights. One participant decoded four minus zero, answering four with practiced eye movements. In their dream, they found themselves in a doctor's office with a large, strange couch in the middle of the room. The lights began to flicker and the participant recognized the Morse code signals transmitting the math problem.[5]

The Dutch group of scientists employed a lucid dream induction technique that was similar to the American team's TLR procedure. Participants practiced eye movements to signal lucidity and answered softly spoken math problems. One subject sat in a car while they received their "assignment." They felt proud when they realized they were dreaming, heard the math problem coming from the car radio, and answered one plus two correctly with eye signals.

The French team observed one twenty-year-old man with narcolepsy, a sleep disorder distinguished by excessive daytime sleepiness and a tendency to lucid dream. Previous work by the French team showed that 78 percent of subjects with narcolepsy are lucid dreamers, which provides a unique opportunity to collect lucid dream episodes within a few naps.[6] The subject reached a lucid dream state easily and had a remarkable ability to control his dreams, reporting an average of four lucid dreams per day. In this study, the subject was asked to respond to various stimuli. He counted the number of times he was tapped on his right hand, distinguished between high- and low-pitch sounds, answered long yes/no questions and identified changes in light. The participant answered by contracting his facial muscles. Two smiles in a row signaled yes while two frowns signaled no.

While the subject knew the types of tasks he might be asked to perform in his sleep, he did not know the specific questions. In one of his lucid dreams, the man was at a party. "I heard your voice as if you were a god," he reported after his nap. "I heard you asking whether I liked chocolate, whether I was studying biology, and whether I speak Spanish." As for the last question, the participant was uncertain how to answer as he didn't speak the language fluently. He decided to answer no and returned to the party.

The scientists had achieved their goal. They had demonstrated that it was possible to communicate with someone in the dream world, and this could be accomplished using sound, light, and touch. Once the researchers had established a connection, subjects were able to process and answer a range of questions using complex thinking.

Interactive Dreaming

IT WAS EASY TO get caught up in the cool factor of these findings. It made me wonder, what were the implications for dream research and for us dreamers? A major challenge of dream research is its reliance on dream recall and dream reporting. Researchers can only study the dreams that people remember and share. Dreams have a tendency to evade our memory. If we don't write them down as soon as we wake up, there's a good chance that we'll forget them. "Interactive dreaming," as it was called in the study, allows researchers to learn about dreams as they happen, sidestepping these challenges.

I thought about a basic idea of scientific investigation. If you wanted to test the effect of an independent variable on a dependent variable, then other factors must be controlled and remain the same. If I wanted to test whether a certain energy drink gave people more energy. Was it the drink that provided the energy boost, or was it the idea of drinking it that caused the change? To test this, I would give two groups of subjects a clear liquid to drink. One group would consume a colourless energy drink while the other group would have water. I would ensure that all other variables remained constant to establish that results weren't caused by other factors.

The same principles hold true for the study of dreams. Say I was investigating the connection between dreams and well-being. If I wanted to test whether a happy dream made people happier during the following day, then I would need to control the content of people's dreams, making one group of subjects dream of happy things while another group did not. Interactive dreaming opens up this possibility.

If scientists can control dreams, they could investigate how the dreaming mind works, testing different cognitive abilities like attention, decision-making, and memory. What complex thought processes are we capable of while dreaming? How do we make decisions in dreams compared to waking life? What types of memory can our dreaming brain access, and how much of our working memory is at our disposal?

Researchers could study how we experience emotions during dreams. Do we feel things the same way in our dreams as in waking life? Emotions are often tempered during the day. Can we exert the same emotional control in our dreams? Studying our dream thoughts, perceptions, and behaviours as they happen offers unique insights into the cognitive dimensions of sleep.

Scientists could explore another level of consciousness through the dreamer's thoughts and experiences.

When I met with Paller, we discussed how interactive dreaming might one day be used to improve our mental health. During the day, we often ruminate over our preoccupations and concerns. One idea is that this negative thought loop carries over to our dreams. Paller described it as a kind of habit formed by our brain. When we fall asleep, this habit might kick in again and cause us to ruminate in our dreams.

This kind of rumination is probably not good for us. What if scientists could cut the process during sleep? Is it possible to cultivate calm sleep, and could this affect our mental health? These big questions are at the edge of research in Paller's lab. Using the principles of TMR, Paller aims to link sounds with calming experiences and create a peaceful mindset during sleep. "This is exactly the non-invasive way that would help people," he said, which would offer a non-pharmacological method to improve psychological well-being.

I was struck by the possibility and promise of dreams as a powerful tool to improve our mental health. Advances in dream science might one day allow us to rewrite upsetting or traumatic memories in our dreams. Maybe interactive dreaming might be used to treat mental health conditions like anxiety, depression, and PTSD. Sounds or other external stimuli could prompt people to practice mindfulness techniques in their dreams and cultivate a calm mindset during sleep.

A New World

WHILE INTERACTIVE DREAMING IS at the forefront of contemporary dream research, lucid dreaming has been around for centuries. In the fourth century BC, the Greek philosopher and scientist Aristotle wrote, "For often, when one is asleep, there is something in consciousness which declares that what then presents itself is but a dream."[7] The first written account of a lucid dream dates back to AD 415 in a letter written by St. Augustine, bishop of Hippo, which is now Annaba, Algeria. The theologian described the dream of Roman physician Gennadius, who was grappling with the possibility of life after death. In the dream, a young man told Gennadius to follow him. The pair came to a city where they heard the most beautiful music. When the physician awoke, he thought of the experience as nothing more than a dream. The next night, he dreamt of the same young man, who asked if Gennadius remembered him. The physician recalled meeting him in the previous night's dream. The young man said, "It is true that you saw these things in sleep, but I would have you know that even now you are seeing in sleep."[8] This prompted Gennadius to realize that he was in a dream. The theologian reflected on his ability to interact with his young dream guide while his sleeping body remained still in bed, offering a new perspective on life after death.

In the eighth century AD, Buddhists in Tibet employed lucid dreaming as a tool for reflection and self-discovery. They practiced specific yoga techniques to sustain awareness in the dream state. Dedicated practice of lucid dreaming enriched waking and dreaming experiences and illuminated the thoughts, emotions, and events of this alternate realm of existence. Tarthang Tulku is a contemporary teacher of Tibetan Buddhism who has written more than thirty books, passing on his wisdom of the spiritual practices. Tulku explores how dream experiences allow us to develop a more flexible attitude and ultimately learn how to change ourselves.

Pioneering dream researcher Marie-Jean-Léon d'Hervey de Saint-Denys was a skilled lucid dreamer who investigated the constructs of his own dream worlds. In his 1867 book *Les Rêves et les Moyens de les Diriger: Observations Pratiques* (Dreams and the Ways to Guide Them: Practical Observations), Saint-Denys shared insights on the dreaming process as well as a self-analysis of his own dream stories. For many months, he worked on gaining awareness of what he called his "true situation," or dream state, until most of his dreams had moments that "kept the feeling of reality."[9]

Then in 1913, lucid dreaming was given its name by Dutch psychiatrist Frederik Willems van Eeden, who conducted rigorous research on the phenomenon. For many years, the physician recorded his dreams. In his collection of 500 reports, he was lucid in more than 350 dreams. He described being asleep while having a full recollection of his daily life as well as having control over his actions. With himself as the subject, van Eeden presented a paper on his own lucid dreams to the Society for Psychical Research. He described the experience of reaching a "state of perfect awareness" in which the dreamer can direct their attention and act freely. "Yet the sleep, as I am able confidently to state, is undisturbed, deep and refreshing."[10]

Eyes Shut Wide

IN THE MID-1970S, THE experiments of two graduate students working continents apart propelled dream research into another dimension. Stephen LaBerge, who is widely considered the contemporary father of lucid dreaming, was a graduate student at Stanford University when he set out to open the lines of communication between the dreaming and waking worlds. At the time, many considered lucid dreaming pseudoscience that didn't warrant rigorous investigation. This didn't deter LaBerge, who knew firsthand the possibility of gaining awareness during the dream state. He'd had lucid dreams since he was five years old and was interested in testing whether it was possible to send a message from a lucid dream to the waking world.

Reflecting on the rapid eye movement that characterizes REM sleep, LaBerge devised a left-right pattern of quick eye movements to signal lucidity. On Friday, January 13, 1978, LaBerge drifted off to sleep in the Stanford lab while Lynn Nagel, the unofficial advisor for his dissertation research, observed from the next room. About seven hours later, LaBerge experienced his first lucid dream in the lab. He was hit by the realization that he must be sleeping because he couldn't see, hear, or feel a thing. He noticed a vacuum manual floating through the air. "It struck me as mere flotsam on the stream of consciousness," wrote LaBerge. As he tried to read the manual, he "had the sensation of opening [his dream] eyes."[11] In his dream, LaBerge moved his finger along an imagined vertical line. His gaze followed his finger up and down, doing the practiced eye movements to signal lucidity. LaBerge became so excited by what he'd accomplished that his thoughts interrupted his dream, which disappeared within seconds.

When LaBerge awoke, he and Nagel identified two pronounced eye movements on his sleep record. LaBerge had sent a message from within his dream, crossing the divide between the waking and dreaming worlds. It took a while to repeat this incredible feat in the lab, which happened in September 1979. Then LaBerge installed a polygraph at home to try and become lucid in a relaxed and familiar environment. Over the course of six weeks, he recorded a dozen additional lucid dreams along with the practiced eye movements signaling awareness.

LaBerge and Nagel submitted their findings for publication and were met with mixed reactions. While one reviewer considered their report excellent and recommended it for publication, another reviewer found it difficult to fathom the possibility of a dreamer experiencing a dream while at the same time signaling the waking world. The reviewer offered ways that LaBerge and Nagel might have come to their "obviously mistaken conclusions."[12] It would take another six months for their paper to be published in *Perceptual and Motor Skills*.

LaBerge learned that he was not the only one sending messages from dreamland. A continent away, another graduate student was conducting similar lucid dreaming experiments. In England, one April night in 1975, Keith Hearne stared bleary-eyed at the polysomnography of Alan Worsley, a practiced lucid dreamer. Hearne had spent the night in the lab at Hull University waiting for the series of eight smooth left-right eye movements to signal lucidity. It was just after 8 a.m. when Hearne witnessed a series of large zigzags scrawled across Worsley's sleep record. It was the message he had been waiting for.

"The signals were coming from another world—the world of dreams—and they were as exciting as if they were emanating from some other solar system in space," explained Hearne. "A channel of communication had been established from the inner universe of the mind in dreaming sleep."[13] Worsley is thought to be the first dreamer to send a signal from the realm of dreams.

To trigger lucidity, Hearne created the Dream Machine. The small device attached to the wrist and sent gentle electric shocks that felt like pinpricks when it detected someone in REM sleep. The dreamer recognized the external stimulus, realized they were dreaming, and signaled lucidity using eye movements. The machine was also a tool to stop nightmares. It could be set at a high respiration rate, a common characteristic of nightmares. When the machine registered accelerated breathing, an alarm sounded to wake the dreamer and put an end to the disturbing dream. Today, Hearne's Dream Machine is on display at London's Science Museum.

In the 1990s, LaBerge developed his own device to encourage lucidity. DreamLight was a sleep mask fitted with lights and sensors to identify eye movements. When the device detected the darting eye movements of REM sleep, the tiny lights flashed from within the sleep mask to signal that the user was in REM. If the user recognized the light cue, they realized that they were in a dream. Now the market is crowded with personal devices that promise lucidity. These include sleep tracking devices to pinpoint REM sleep, when most lucid dreams occur, sleep masks with customizable LED lights and sounds to prompt awareness, and apps to practice lucid dream induction techniques. There are many high-tech and low-tech tools designed to promote lucidity. See the Dreamer's Toolkit at the back of the book for some tips that I gathered from dream scientists and practiced lucid dreamers.

How to Build a Dream

TODAY, NEUROIMAGING STUDIES ALLOW scientists to explore the brain activity of this rare and transient dream experience. I was curious to learn what happens in the brain when we begin to poke holes in our dream plots and realize that everything around us is a construct of our dreaming brain. What are the mental mechanics that allow us to take control of our dreams? I sat down with cognitive neuroscientist Bejamin Baird to find out.

Baird's main interest is consciousness and using science to better understand the nature of reality. Spontaneous states like dreaming and mind-wandering offer some interesting insights into the dynamics of consciousness. Lucid dreaming is another realm that provides a unique opportunity to study awareness and self-reflection in the dream state.

In 2004, Baird was introduced to lucid dreaming as an undergraduate at the University of Texas in Austin, where he is currently a research professor of cognitive neuroscience. He was up late one night surfing the internet and came across the Lucidity Institute, which was founded by LaBerge. Baird had been fascinated by consciousness since he was fourteen, and he had never considered the possibility of reaching this level of consciousness while asleep. "It blew my mind," he said. He fell asleep thinking about such an exciting prospect. That night, Baird had his first lucid dream.

He found himself in a house with his friend's dog Murray, a gentle Boston terrier. In the dream, Murray was being uncharacteristically aggressive, biting Baird, which didn't make sense. Then Baird discovered that he had an odd number of fingers, which tipped him off that he was dreaming. The first thing that he thought to do was go outside and try to fly. As he soared through the sky, everything went black and he woke up.

During the day, we are constantly using our episodic memory. While we spend a lot of mental energy focusing on physical and mental tasks, our thoughts tend to drift, taking us away from the moment. When our brain is in mind-wandering mode, it's only a matter of time before our thoughts drift to things that have happened in the past or plans for the future. "We're constantly in this episodic flow of this narrative self-consciousness in which we're embedded in time," Baird said. He began to wonder if spontaneous, self-reflective thinking carried over to sleep and dreams. What happens when we gain awareness in a lucid dream? Do we focus only on the excitement of the moment, or do we reflect on the past and the future? Baird decided to find out.

A few years ago, while working as a research scientist at the University of Wisconsin-Madison, Baird studied spontaneous thoughts in waking, NREM sleep, and REM sleep. The idea was to test whether autobiographical memory carried over to sleep and dreams. They recruited 138 subjects and brought them into the lab. The first task was to have participants focus on a fixed spot for half an hour. About once every minute, a sound played and subjects were asked to describe any images, thoughts, or feelings that were going through their minds. They slept in the lab and were woken during Stage 2 and REM sleep at different points throughout the night. Again, the subjects were asked to describe their thoughts. Were they reflecting on the memory of a past experience, an experience that they had forgotten the details of, or no experience at all?

Baird discovered that self-reflective thoughts of the past and the future happened rarely during Stage 2 and REM sleep. In more than 3,500 dream reports, only about 1 percent of thoughts used episodic memory. This was in stark contrast to what they found when subjects were awake. When they stared at a fixed point, their thoughts drifted to past memories or plans for the future 25 percent of the time.[14]

It is common to dream about what is happening in our waking lives. We carry our waking preoccupations and concerns with us into our dreams. We might even dream about an event that happened in the past. But here's the catch. It's the reflective thought process that is missing in ordinary dreams. We might weave details from an episodic memory into our dreams. But we don't hit the replay button on an entire episodic memory. And we don't make plans to reach our future goals. The story takes an interesting turn when you look at lucid dreams, which usually happen during REM sleep.

In lucid dreams, people reflect on their past as well as plan for the future. It could be something they want to try in their dreams like practice a skill or work through a problem. "My view is that you're de-embedded from this episodic self in ordinary dreams. You don't have the context," said Baird. "But when you become lucid, you get that back." One idea is that the level of consciousness during a lucid dream is more akin to waking consciousness than the altered state in ordinary dreams.

The Lucid Brain

WHAT HAPPENS IN THE brain when we gain awareness and possibly control of our dreams? In REM sleep, brain activity fluctuates, with peaks and valleys of activity. Lucid dreams tend to happen when the brain is most activated during REM. As we move from NREM into this final stage of the sleep cycle, our respiration, eye movements, and heart rate pick up speed.

Brain scans show there are certain regions involved with lucid dreaming.

A functional magnetic resonance imaging (fMRI) is a type of imaging that measures activity in different parts of the brain by monitoring blood flow in different areas. This lets scientists understand what is happening in the brain when we are busy doing different activities during the day as well as in our sleep and dreams. One major hurdle, though, is getting subjects to sleep in an MRI machine, which can be claustrophobic and noisy.

One fMRI study showed increased activity in the prefrontal cortex during lucid dreams in REM sleep.[15] This frontal brain region, which is associated with complex thinking like logic, reason, and control, is normally quiet during REM sleep. Yet lucid dreamers are self-aware. They can make decisions and carry out predetermined plans, which fits with the results from the fMRI study.

Now to put this in the context of reflective thinking during lucid dreams. Functional neuroimaging studies have shown that retrieving episodic memories involves the prefrontal cortex.[16] This area is quiet during REM sleep. And lucid dreams, which occur mostly during this sleep stage, involve high-level thinking that is associated with the prefrontal cortex. Putting all of this together, it makes sense that lucid dreaming, which is characterized by self-reflective thinking, is associated with increased activation in frontal regions of the brain, while the same frontal areas are quiet during ordinary dreams, which don't usually involve the same level of self-awareness.

A recent study from a team of researchers in the Netherlands found some differences in the frequencies in certain brain regions during lucid dreaming in REM compared to non-lucid REM sleep. It appears that lucid dreaming is different from waking consciousness as well as from ordinary dreaming. Yet with limited neuroimaging data, scientists are just beginning to understand what exactly is happening in the brain during a lucid dream and when increased brain activity occurs along the journey to full lucidity.

It's interesting how many of us can gain awareness while remaining immersed in our dreams. Approximately 23 percent of people have at least one lucid dream a month while 55 percent of people have experienced at least one lucid dream in their lifetime.[16] Doing reality checks can help people realize they are in a dream. Sometimes the numbers on a clock are distorted or the time is illogical in a dream. Your dream-self could try to count your fingers. Seeing an odd number might tip you off that things aren't quite right.

To complicate matters, lucidity can be fleeting and fickle. It can seem next to impossible to hold onto awareness in the dream state. Whenever I realize that I'm dreaming, I'm easily distracted if something exciting or terrifying happens, and I let myself be carried away by my dream.

What if there was a way to up our chances of having a lucid dream? What if we could enhance brain activation during REM sleep and increase the odds of becoming lucid? Early work by LaBerge showed that neural activation during REM is driven predominantly by acetylcholine. This neurotransmitter is involved in memory, attention, and learning. In 2018, Baird, LaBerge, and clinical psychologist Kristen LaMarca tested whether driving up acetylcholine to increase activation during REM would help to induce lucid dreaming as well as influence dream recall and dream content.

For the study, they gathered 121 subjects with an interest in lucid dreaming. The participants were trained in LaBerge's Mnemonic Induction of Lucid Dreams (MILD) technique to induce lucid dreaming. MILD provides strategies to help people recognize when they are in a dream in order to become lucid.

Participants spent three nights in the lab. They awoke four-and-a-half hours after they went to bed and remained awake for thirty minutes. Subjects remembered a dream and worked at memorizing it. Divided into three groups, the subjects were randomly given either 0 millligrams, 4 milligrams, or 8 milligrams of galantamine. This fast-acting medication increases acetylcholine, which drives up brain activity during REM sleep. The idea was to test whether this increased brain activity would increase lucid dreaming. Then participants returned to bed, where they did some MILD techniques until they fell back asleep. Waking people up in the night allowed the team to study two forms of lucid dreaming: dream-initiated lucid dreams that arise during a dream and wake-initiated lucid dreams that happen from the waking state.

The results were remarkable. Approximately 27 percent of participants who took 4 milligrams of galantamine reported at least one lucid dream. There was a sharp spike in lucid dreams for people who were given the higher dose of galantamine. Approximately 42 percent of participants who took 8 milligrams of galantamine had at least one lucid dream. In subjects who were given a placebo, only 14 percent had a lucid dream. This is a massive effect, said Baird, which offers a major clue to understanding the neurobiology of dreaming.

Researchers spend countless hours waiting for subjects to become lucid in the lab so they can study dreams from within. It is difficult for novice as well as practiced lucid dreamers to become lucid when they are being observed. It is even more challenging for subjects to become lucid when they are sleeping in an MRI machine so that researchers can study brain activity during a lucid dream. Galantamine could increase people's chances of having lucid dreams in the lab, which opens up the possibility of getting more data on this unique dream state.

Dream Big

BAIRD AND I TALKED about some of the ways people can use this powerful experience to improve their waking lives. With limitless abilities and resources, lucid dreamers could rethink nagging problems that seem unsolvable during the day or practice a new skill that they are trying to master. A ballplayer might adjust his bat until he was able to knock the ball out of the park, while a pianist's hands could repeat a chord progression until it became ingrained, and her fingers flew across the black-and-white keys. In this way, lucid dreams become a kind of training ground to test out variations and learn from different responses. "That could be transformational, especially if practiced over time," said Baird.

I discovered several studies that found lucid dreaming to be an effective treatment to reduce nightmares among people with chronic and recurrent nightmares. While there are limited studies, the findings are promising. One day, lucid dreaming might offer an alternative treatment for mental health conditions like anxiety or PTSD. With the guidance of a clinician, lucid dreamers could rewrite upsetting or traumatic memories, helping them to escape the deep grooves of the same unhelpful thought processes.

"You're able to engage with the psychological content in the dream while it's happening," said Baird, who suggested that real magic happens when you work with a qualified clinician and gain the therapeutic benefit. Lucid dreaming offers another kind of transformational experience that can change how we think, feel, and behave.

Lucid dreaming can also be used as a creative tool. It offers a unique combination of focus and freedom of thought that generates new perspectives and inspiration. Baird told me about a composer in New York City who writes music in his lucid dreams. His technique is to search his dreams for a room with a radio. When he switches on the radio, symphonies begin to play. He listens to the music that is a creation of his own mind. The man wakes up and transcribes the symphonies, composing his dream inspiration onto the page. Artists who are practiced lucid dreamers could imagine a door that opens into an art gallery, said Baird. Setting this expectation, the lucid dreamers could walk into a gallery of paintings that their dreaming brain had created.

Before he answered math problems from his dreams, Mazurek came across some of LaBerge's writing on the experience of lucid dreaming. He told me how impactful LaBerge's writing was on him. Mazurek paraphrased a question posed by LaBerge: imagine what it would be like to control the other half of your existence. We spend a large portion of our lives asleep. For a good chunk of this time, we explore the dream world. A world that is usually out of our control, which Mazurek views as a loss. "The power of intentionally dreaming, of lucid dreaming, even just being aware of what's going on in your dreams, is a way of reclaiming that other half of our existence that a lot of people leave on the table. That's why I find dreams so fascinating," he said. Then with a grin, Mazurek added, "Also, it's really cool to fly."

In labs around the world, dream scientists are working on ways to guide our dreams. They are using sensations like sound, touch, and smell to connect with dreamers and flag specific dream content. For my next adventure in dreamland, I tried my own at-home experiment. I tested a simple dream engineering tool that helped me guide my dreams and understand a powerful message from a collective of artists, scientists, and dream engineers: "Dreams change us. We change dreams."

Chapter Twelve

DREAM ENGINEERING: THE NEXT FRONTIER

I WAS A WRITER ON ASSIGNMENT, AND I WAS BEING SENT TO MY most remote location yet. One humid summer afternoon, I travelled to the border between the waking and dreaming worlds, the time zone where thoughts and images tumbled into each other, transforming into the wild and wonderful stuff that dreams are made of. I ventured into sleep onset, the first few minutes of sleep that are so light I could still hear the kids giggling and shrieking as they ran through the icy water of a sprinkler a few backyards over.

As my tired body settled into bed, my mind sifted through memories from the day. It's thought that during the first few minutes of sleep, our brain tags certain memories to revisit later in the night. I wondered which thoughts and experiences would make their way into my dreams. This is a natural process that happens to all of us. But what if we don't want to leave our dreams to chance? What if we want certain thoughts to jump the queue and get front-of-the-line priority to shape our dreams?

For more than five thousand years, people have used different waking rituals and practices to dream about a chosen topic, a technique known as dream incubation. To achieve this purpose, from ancient Egypt and Greece to India, North Africa, and Australia, people have practiced fasting, bathing in cold water, or sleeping in a temple, shrine, or cave. Some people sought knowledge while others looked for spiritual enlightenment or healing. Cures included rest, exercise, eating figs and ashes from a god's altar, or being suspended upside down.[1] Today, the sacred practice continues for many societies and religions around the world. This includes Indigenous peoples who value dreams as sources of guidance, knowledge, and creative inspiration.

What's new, and what I set out to investigate, is Targeted Dream Incubation (TDI), which uses external stimuli to connect with a dreamer and encourage them to focus on a particular topic or theme. Adam Haar and reseaarchers from MIT and Harvard University developed this contemporary incubation method using sound and touch to reach a dreamer as they traversed through sleep onset, moving from waking to sleep. These first few minutes of sleep are characterized by hypnagogia, dreamy thoughts and images that are often related to recent waking experiences. As a montage of images, thoughts, and sensations flooded a person's mind, a voice recording prompted them to focus on a chosen topic.

TDI is part of the emerging field of dream engineering that uses technology to connect with dreamers and help them guide their dreams. Just as sounds or other stimuli are employed to boost memory consolidation during sleep or help dreamers become lucid, this novel technique uses stimuli to guide people's thoughts as they drift off with the hope of influencing their dreams. It is well-established that we often dream about experiences from earlier in the day, and the thoughts that swirl around our heads as we fall asleep can influence our dreams. Research shows that if we are ruminating over negative thoughts during sleep onset, it's more likely that we will have bad dreams later in the night. The loop of negative thoughts even makes our sleep quality worse. As I pulled the blinds, silenced my phone, and prepared for my makeshift dream experiment, I wondered how difficult it would be to forget about what was on my mind and guide my dream thoughts.

"Remember to Think of a Tree"

IT WAS MIDAFTERNOON ON a humid July day when I attempted my first dream incubation session. I was travelling to the elusive and short-lived period of sleep onset to investigate whether I could choose a waking thought, hold on to it, and carry it with me into those first few minutes of sleep. The blazing sun illuminated the edges of my closed bedroom blinds. The air was heavy and still. I lay on top of my duvet, flopping back and forth as I tried to find a comfortable position. I hadn't been sleeping well. This was a cruel irony considering that I was spending most of my waking hours thinking about the importance of dreams. "Sleep can't be forced. Just allowed," explained Haar in an instructional video that I watched before I began my dream experiment.

I had chatted with Haar several times, and he kindly agreed to help me set up my own TDI session. The dream researcher made it very simple and low-tech. First, I picked a topic to think about. In the TDI study, Haar had subjects incubate on the theme of a tree, so that was what I chose to try and dream about. Then I recorded a voice prompt that would play as soon as I closed my eyes, telling me to keep the intended thought in my mind. Once I moved from drowsiness to light sleep, the recording would replay to focus my dreamy thoughts on trees. I recorded a different prompt that would play once I had been in light sleep for a few more minutes. OK. I could do this. I just had to relax and let my mind drift.

With my laptop beside me on the bed, I hit the start button and began my first of five guided naps. As I slid on my eye mask and settled in, a recording of my voice told me to "remember to think of a tree." Images of different trees flashed through my mind like a stack of cue cards. There was the lilac tree in my backyard. The forsythia tree that had lost its vibrant yellow flowers. The maple tree in front of our house that wouldn't seem to grow. None of these images kept my attention. Oh, wait. What about the cedars along the back of our yard? They were eight feet tall now, but I pictured them as tiny saplings. We had transplanted them from the woods behind the log cabin that my husband's family used to own. It was a way of holding on to the cabin after it was sold.

My mind flooded with memories of our time at the cabin. Playing cards by the warmth of the wood stove. Bursting out into the refreshing cold for our midnight walk on Christmas Eve. The sound of snow crunching beneath our boots as we followed the narrow, winding road through the trees, our path illuminated by the moon. A pile of us tobogganing down the hill from the cabin, our laughter echoing through the valley. I had a quick intermission from my thoughts as I registered the monotone beeping sound of a truck backing up outside my house. Within seconds, I was back at the cabin. I imagined those sweltering summer nights when we tried to sleep on the screened porch while a symphony of cicadas played around us. I could still feel the stillness of the place, surrounded by darkness, with no one around for miles.

A recording of my voice interrupted my thoughts and reminded me to think of a tree. I tried to stay focused on the idea of a tree while I let my mind roam. It was a kind of mental see-saw as my mind focused and let go over and over again. It reminded me of story meetings at a magazine where I used to work. I'd brainstorm story ideas with other writers and editors. We would try to stay on track, but inevitably our conversations would get carried away. Some of the best ideas came when we veered off in different directions.

Haar said that the verbal prompts weren't intended to wake me up. They wouldn't let me fall into a deep sleep, either. This delicate balance allowed me to maintain awareness of the strange thoughts that kept popping into my head. OK. Focus. Think of a tree.

Oh, wait. There was that willow tree. I had almost forgotten about it. It must have been twenty years ago when Dimitri and I planted a cutting from a willow tree beside the cabin's circular gravel driveway, and against all odds, it grew. It grew so tall that it began to bend toward the other side of the narrow driveway, creating a lush, green archway to drive under. This reminded me of a horseshoe. In my mind, I threw the horseshoe across the valley, into the woods. Haar had said to "enjoy the changes that sleeping creates in your thought patterns," so I just went with it. I was transported back to the day that Dimitri and I got lost in the forest for hours, turning ourselves around until every tree looked the same. While I was in the in-between world of sleep onset, something strange happened. As I imagined myself standing in the forest, staring at the thick, twisted tree branches, the branches scooped me up and placed me on top of the canopy of trees. I could see the cabin. It was so close. I couldn't believe it. How could we have been so lost that day?

I moved up and down with the sway of the trees, and the canopy became an ocean. The water was so dark it appeared black. I wondered what was underneath me as I moved along with the waves. I grabbed fistfuls of water, and the tips of my fingers grazed something. I grabbed hold and pulled it out of the water and discovered that it was the roots of a tree. I wondered if this is what I was supposed to be thinking of. Do roots count? Or did it need be the entire tree? I remembered Haar saying that it was OK to think abstractly about a tree. My thoughts could shift and change. It didn't need to be a concrete idea.

One image tumbled into another until I found myself lying on the grass in front of my childhood home. It was cool in the shade of the birch tree, and I watched the leaves flutter in the breeze. Somehow, I was wearing my kid-sized Snoopy PJs. They used to be my absolute favourite, and I focused on them for a bit. Woodstock was perched on Snoopy's nose. Oh, how I loved those PJs. I refocused my internal camera and took a wide shot of myself lying on the grass. I thought of the tree roots beneath me. The roots became veins that began to pump with blood, full of life. Then they broke through the earth and enveloped me. But I wasn't scared. I didn't get the feeling that I was being suffocated. It was more like the comfort of a strong hug. Then the root-veins broke through the ground underneath my old house and lifted it into the sky. The house landed in my backyard where I now live. My parents walked out of the house with my mom wearing her now-vintage massive red glasses. Then the scene evaporated when my recorded voice asked, "Tell me, what were you thinking about?"

So it worked. I dreamt of a tree. Many trees, actually, and the images of cedars, pines, and birches made me think of memories that I had long forgotten. Places and events from another time.

Night Shift

I WAS EXCITED TO tell Haar about my experience and get his take on it. I told him it reminded me of a dreamy brainstorming session. This led us to a discussion about the similarities and differences between dreaming and mind-wandering, or daydreaming. The brain's default mode network (DMN) is activated when our mind wanders from whatever we're doing and we stare off into space, often reflecting on past events or future plans. Most components of the brain's DMN are active during REM sleep. In fact, G. William Domhoff and Kieran Fox suggest that dreaming, specifically during REM, is an "intensified form of mind-wandering."[2] One difference is that during mind-wandering, we get wrapped up in personal concerns and emotions, while the immersive nature of dreams centres around a simulated version of ourselves and a "here and now" feeling.[3]

Sleep onset is this in-between space that bridges waking and sleep. Although it lasts only a few minutes, there is so much going on. I thought about how most nights my mind shuffles through thoughts and concerns from the day. The concreteness of these thoughts then begins to soften. Thoughts become malleable. It's a gradual process of shifting semantically, of losing your sense of time, your sense of body or sense of self, said Haar. There is this beautiful cascading breakdown into dreaming, he added. Yet at the same time, we maintain some cognitive control.

It's the in-between nature of sleep onset that fascinates Haar. In this mixed state, it's like being partly awake and partly asleep. It's a time and place where brain activity changes bit by bit and you lose parts of your brain function. I thought about the sensation of being woken up after a few minutes of sleep. It always made me feel groggy and out of synch as whispers of strange, dreamy thoughts linger in my mind.

I pictured sleep onset as a mash up of sleeping and waking, daydreaming and brainstorming. In those first few minutes of sleep, we loosen our grip on the external world while our thoughts tumble together in a dreamy brainstorming session until thoughts become images, and these images become dream experiences. By studying this in between, scientists are also learning about other states of consciousness and how they fit together on our continuum of thought and experience.

"I like the in between because it's poetic and weird," said Haar. "It's just right at your fingertips and it's, I think, worthwhile to occupy in betweens when people have told you there's either here or there." We talked about how each of us creates our own world in which to live. These worlds are influenced by the inner world that we prioritize. Some of us might focus on gratitude while others might focus on intentional, task-oriented thinking to guide our days and shape our lives. "If we focus on clothes, we notice clothes. If we focus on cars, our memories, our attention, our conversations all shift to cars," explained Haar. "We set our filters and expectations and then slowly we become them."

What if we choose to prioritize our dreams? What if, instead of focusing on what's logical and rational in our waking lives, we concentrate on the bizarre, creative thoughts that our dreaming brain connects in new and unique ways? Like when something from yesterday is somehow connected to a memory from your childhood. This sparks new perspectives and creative insights.

Many artists have found creative inspiration in their dreams. Paul McCartney awoke with the melody for "Yesterday" fully formed in his mind. Keith Richards woke up in the night with his legendary guitar riff for "(I Can't Get No) Satisfaction" in his head. He recorded the riff and the famous line, "I can't get no satisfaction" on a cassette recorder before dozing off again.

If we pay attention to the bizarre and strange dream thoughts floating in the periphery, then maybe we will be more attuned to what is unique in the outside world. Maybe we will be more equipped to make something that is novel.

"I think it's pretty clear that everyone has the capacity for this kind of thinking. But many people overlook it," said Haar. "Part of my big excitement is, if they quit overlooking it, it would really make an artist out of everyone, depending on what you mean by artist." We get to decide what creativity and art look like, for each of us.

Brainstorm

IT'S THE COMBINATION OF free thinking and awareness of spontaneous thought that makes the first stage of sleep a natural sleep-induced brainstormer of creative insights and ideas. A few years ago, a study led by cognitive scientist Célia Lacaux showed that spending fifteen seconds in Stage 1 sleep almost tripled the possibility of having a creative insight into a math problem.[4] Subjects were given eight numbers and asked to find a final number as quickly as possible. They were told that using two simple rules would guide them to the solution. Little did they know, there was a hidden rule that would help them solve the problem much faster. After studying the math task, subjects were given a twenty-minute break to relax in a dark room. As they lay in a semi-reclined chair with their eyes closed, the subjects held a bottle in their right hand. If they drifted off and dropped the bottle, they were asked to share their thoughts.

This technique was inspired by the napping routine of inventor Thomas Edison, who used to drift off while holding a sphere. If the object fell to the ground, the noise would waken him, allowing the inventor to record any dreamy creative ideas. This brings us back to Salvador Dalí and his "slumber with a key" method for creative inspiration. As he drifted off, Dalí would focus on a problem that was weighing on his mind. As sleep took hold, the key would slip from his grasp, fall onto a plate below, and wake him so he could record his surreal ideas.

In this more recent study, the subjects were divided into three groups: the Stage 1 group that had at least one thirty-second period of Stage 1 yet didn't have any deeper sleep stage, the wake group that stayed awake for their twenty-minute break, and the Stage 2 group that had at least one thirty-second period of Stage 2 sleep. Approximately 83 percent of the Stage 1 group gained a creative insight compared to 30 percent of the wake group and about 14 percent of the Stage 2 group. Lacaux and her fellow researchers concluded that sleep onset is a "creative sweet spot" to generate creative insights compared to staying awake. If we keep sleeping and fall deeper into Stage 2 sleep, we don't benefit from the same creative boost.

Haar and a group of reasearchers tested whether incubating a topic in Stage 1 sleep affected waking creativity. They used their TDI method to determine whether incubating a certain theme in Stage 1 enhanced waking creative performance more than Stage 1 sleep alone.[5] Subjects were asked to incubate on a tree. Unlike my low-tech, at-home experiment, the study used a sleep tracking device called Dormio, which was invented by Haar in collaboration with scientists at MIT and Harvard. The concept and creation of Dormio were part of Haar's master's degree and PhD at MIT.

The market is crowded with sleep trackers. An interesting feature of Dormio is its live sleep staging. Most off-the-shelf trackers give only a summary of data for a sleep report, averaging out data from across the night. Dormio's high-quality sensors provide live data across the cycle, allowing for more precise analysis. Dormio is a wearable device with a band around the wrist that is connected by wires to small bands around the index and middle fingers. The device is fitted with sensors that identify changes in heart rate, muscle tone, and perspiration as someone enters sleep onset. Dormio is connected to an app where a user records verbal cues to guide dream thoughts. At certain times, these recordings are played to prompt the user to think of a specific theme and then later on report what they were thinking about.

For the study, forty-nine subjects had an afternoon nap in the lab. There were four randomly selected groups: the sleep incubation, sleep no-incubation, wake incubation, and wake no-incubation groups. Here's how it worked for the two sleep groups: One to five minutes after Dormio identified Stage 1 sleep, an audio prompt was played. The difference was in the message. For the sleep incubation group, the recording asked subjects to "remember to think of a tree," while the sleep no-incubation group was told to "remember to observe your thoughts."[6]

The protocol was a bit different for the wake groups. Those in the wake incubation group were encouraged to let their mind wander for about seven to twelve minutes. After each period, the subjects gave a verbal report and were then told to "continue thinking about a tree." The wake no-incubation group followed the same protocol as the wake group except they were asked to observe their thoughts rather than think of a tree.

The results were remarkable, highlighting the creative nature of Stage 1 sleep. The researchers examined the impact of incubation on people's dreams. In the sleep incubation group, 70 percent of dream reports directly referred to the theme of a tree. This was lower for the wake incubation group at 52 percent of daydream reports about a tree. The results were very differ-ent for the subjects who didn't incubate on the specific topic. For the sleep no-incubation group, only one participant reported a dream about a tree. For the wake no-incubation group, there were no daydream reports of a tree.

Next, the researchers investigated whether incubation affected waking creative performance. To test this, subjects completed three assessments that measured different types of creative performance once they awoke from their nap. There was the Creative Storytelling Task that had subjects write a creative story that contained "tree." The Alternative Uses Task had subjects list any creative, alternative uses for a tree that they could imagine. For the Verb Generation Task, participants were given thirty-one nouns related to a tree (for example, forest, branch, and leaf) and asked to provide the first associated verb that they could think of for each noun.

In terms of creativity, both sleep groups outperformed the wake groups. This aligned with previous findings that sleep is an optimal envi-ronment for creative ideas. It also supported Lacaux's findings that sleep onset is an "ideal cocktail for creativity."[7] The sleep incubation group had a significantly higher creativity score than all of the other groups, including the waking subjects who incubated on the theme of a tree. This showed that incubation along with Stage 1 provided the most creative benefits.

Then they looked at the relationship between frequency of an incubated theme and creativity. The subjects who dreamt the most about a tree had the greatest creative boost in relation to the incubated theme. They came up with more creative stories about a tree, thought of more creative, alternative uses for a tree, and had more semantic distance between "tree" and alterna-tive uses of the word. This reflected the idea that a greater semantic distance between associated words is linked to higher creativity. For example, "flut-tered" and "tree" have more semantic distance than "leaves" and "tree."

"This is as close as we have come to a controlled experiment suggesting causal links between dream content and post-sleep cognition," explained Haar, adding, "The door is open to better and bigger experiments linking dreams with memory, emotion, and learning."

Stream of Altered Consciousness

WHY WOULD MORE TREES in our dreams make us more creative about the idea of trees? In the study of creativity, there is the concept of the associative theory.[8] It's about rearranging ideas and thoughts that are already associated in our mind to create new combinations. The more remote the ideas are within these new combinations, the more creative the result. The thinking is, if we're able to make these fresh and new associations, we're able to come up with more creative ideas. We've got to have enough cognitive control to be aware of and reflect on these creative ideas, which is exactly what sleep onset provides.

During these first few minutes of sleep, our mind wanders and we stray from our waking logical and analytical paths of thought, which gives us the cognitive flexibility to pair up remote ideas and generate new, creative insights. This reflects Robert Stickgold and Antonio Zandra's recent model on a possible function of dreaming called NEXTUP, which stands for network exploration to understand possibilities.[9] NEXTUP looks at the abstract associations we make between memories while we sleep. By exploring and strengthening weak and overlooked associations, we gain new knowledge and insights.

This is what happened during my at-home incubation session. After I'd finished my naps, I sat down at my desk to type out the scribbled, disjointed notes about my dream thoughts. The first references were concrete images of trees that came to mind easily. I thought of the different types of trees around my house that I see every day. Somewhere along the way, I began to think of distant memories that involved trees. From here, my mind drifted to other loosely associated memories, like the times at the log cabin or the countless hours I lay under the birch in front of my childhood home.

As I drifted deeper into sleep onset, these associations became more remote and creative. Some of the trees were personified, their branches like strong arms lifting me high above the forest where I was lost. Or they became the vein-like roots pulsing with blood and wrapping me in a strong hug. Haar explained that the deeper you get into sleep onset, the more bizarre and dreamlike your thoughts become. This is when time gets stirred up and memories mix together in strange new ways. One day I'd like to repeat the experiment and include a creative assessment to measure my waking creativity.

The experiment reminded me of the connection between the waking and dreaming worlds. It's well established that our dreaming mind is connected to our sleeping body. This made me think of how I incorporate the tedious beeping of my alarm into a dream so I can keep sleeping a little while longer. More than 175 years ago, dream scientists were testing the power of this connection. In Saint-Denys's pioneering dream experiments, he used scent to show how external stimuli can conjure associated memories that influence our dreams. Also recall Alfred Maury's guillotine dream had him imagine his head being severed by a guillotine as his headboard fell onto his neck while he slept.

Haar and I discussed how we have multiple lines of cognition working at the same time, even in our sleep. Lucid dreamers can recognize the voice of the experimenter telling them to move their eyes. During my incubation session, I noticed a truck's high-pitched back-up alarm while I followed the thread of my dreamy thoughts of trees. Our attention can be in several places at once without us knowing it. We talked about a classic example in the neuroscience of attention that is known as the cocktail party problem. We often think that we're totally focused on a particular task or conversation. Imagine I'm chatting with someone at a party as I balance a wine glass and napkin of tiny canapes. While I'm in the middle of telling this person that I had the weirdest dream about trees, someone across the room says my name. Or maybe they say an emotionally charged word like murder. My head whips in their direction to see what's happening. Little did I know that I was processing the words at the same time I was telling my story. I just wasn't bringing the words into first order consciousness and awareness.

Haar thinks that something similar happens during sleep onset. When it comes to attention, "I think you're making a lot of choices," he said. While I was floating above the trees, I also noticed the beeping sound of the truck in case it was something that I needed to attend to. It wasn't my main focus. Yet it was still within my grasp of awareness, floating somewhere in the background. During sleep onset, there are so many different arms or kinds of "tendrils of cognition" happening at once, said Haar.

As I tried to think about trees, my attention was also being interrupted by some performance anxiety. I wanted the experiment to work, which naturally made me worry that it wouldn't. Haar said nervousness and stress can keep us awake. But the more naps that I had, the more I was able to tune out the external world and let my thoughts drift. Haar suggested that the more you notice the strange thoughts and images of hypnagogia, the more you can choose to stay with them, and guide them. Then you can get better at following the multiple streams of attention by gently suggesting something to yourself and then backing off to see where it goes. "It's really a learned skill, which is cool," he said with a smile.

Dream Guide

IN CONTEMPORARY SCIENCE, A well-known study highlighted the potential of dream incubation as a problem-solving tool. I spoke with Harvard dream researcher Deirdre Barrett to learn about her 1993 study. Seventy-six college students were asked to choose a real problem in their life that they were motivated to solve. The problem had to be objective so that anyone could agree on a correct answer. Yet there could be many possible answers to the problem. Some students selected homework problems while other problems were practical. One student couldn't reconfigure the furniture in their new apartment so that the smaller living space would fit a large cedar chest.

The students came up with a simple phrase to represent the problem and repeated it to themselves at bedtime, forming an image of the problem in their mind's eye, said Barrett. If they couldn't visualize it, they placed a photo or object representing the problem beside their bed, staring at it before they fell asleep. The students incubated a dream about their chosen problem for one week or until they dreamt of a suitable solution. They kept a dream journal, indicating which dreams related to their chosen problem, if there were any attempts to solve the dilemma, and if so, if there was a satisfactory solution.

Barrett had the subjects as well as independent judges rate whether any dreams were about their problem, and if they came up with a solution in one or more of their dreams. The subjects and the judges rated 50 percent of dreams as containing content about the problem. When it came to solving the problem in their dreams, the judges rated that one-quarter of dreams accomplished this, while subjects felt that one-third came up with a suitable solution. "The dreamers were endorsing some that were more metaphoric," said Barrett, which let them come up with a concrete solution if they thought about the dream and what it might imply.[10] The student with the new apartment couldn't figure out how to arrange their bedroom to fit the cedar chest. In their dream, they came up with the creative solution to use the chest as a coffee table in the living room. Until the dream, they'd only thought of the chest as a piece of bedroom furniture.

Another student had applied to two clinical psychology and two industrial psychology programs and couldn't decide which to choose. The student dreamt of flying over a map of the United States. In the dream, the pilot said there was a problem with the engine and they needed to find a safe place to land. As they hovered over the student's home state, the pilot announced that the entire state was dangerous. The student awoke and realized that the two clinical psychology programs were in the state where she grew up and her parents still lived. The industrial programs were located in Texas and California. The student realized that it was more important to choose a school based on location away from home rather than the type of psychology program. Interestingly, the students in the study came up with solutions that they had not been consciously aware of.

Today, technology allows dream scientists to use tools like Dormio to target different sleep stages and attempt to influence dreams across the night. Beyond incubating on a certain topic for creative inspiration or problem solving, dream engineering techniques aim to rewrite nightmares, facilitate lucid dreaming, consolidate memories, and boost learning. This is done using different kinds of external stimuli, like sound, smell, or touch, which are introduced at certain stages in the sleep cycle.

Dream engineering is now moving beyond the lab as scientists design apps and other tools that we can use at home. Haar and his MIT lab mate Tomás Vega launched the Dust app, which is translating this exciting dream research into products for the public. Its tag line encompasses the power and possibility of dream engineering: "We change dreams. Dreams change us." Dust has several programs to choose from. You can focus on improving dream recall, incubate on a chosen dream topic, or work on reducing nightmares and stress dreams. Look for the app and see if you can guide your dreams.

Dream engineering continues to expand the bounds of dream research. In Ken Paller's lab at Northwestern University, scientists are investigating strategies that could change brain activity to create a positive experience. Currently, they are linking sound with calming experiences to reactivate a positive and relaxed frame of mind during sleep. If we ruminate during the day, there is a good possibility that we ruminate during sleep. This new research aims to cultivate calm sleep.

Something as innocuous as a bad smell can leave such a lasting impression on the sleeping brain that it may curb an addictive habit. A 2014 study tested whether odour emitted during sleep could curb smoking. While subjects were in Stage 2 and REM sleep, the odour of rotten eggs was released along with the smell of a cigarette. Associating this bad odour with cigarettes reduced smoking among participants over the following week. There was an even greater and prolonged reduction in smoking when subjects were exposed to the associated odours in Stage 2 sleep compared to REM sleep. After exposure during Stage 2, subjects smoked 30 percent fewer cigarettes the following week. There was no reduction in smoking when the combined odours were presented during waking.[11]

It can be very difficult to quit smoking, with many people relapsing and trying to quit several times. It would be interesting to see if the subjects were still smoking less in the long term. The study highlighted how new associations learned during sleep might alter addictive habits. But what if a cognitive prompt was used to enhance a behaviour like shopping, playing video games, or drinking?

Advertising in Dreamland

IN 2021, AFTER MORE than three decades of being shut out from broadcasting ads during the Super Bowl, Molson Coors launched an advertising campaign in the world of dreams. While Anheuser-Busch InBev enjoyed its advertising deal with the Super Bowl, Molson Coors publicized what it called its own dream incubation experiment to influence people's dreams. Numerous social media users participated along with singer-songwriter Zayn Malik. "When Coors asked me if they could induce a refreshing dream while I sleep for you all to watch on Instagram Live, I thought . . . well that *is* very strange. So of course, I said yes," said Malik. "It's been a minute since I've had a good night's sleep, so let's see if it works. I love a good science project."[12]

In the nights leading up to Super Bowl Sunday, people were instructed to watch a ninety-second video clip of snow-covered mountains, waterfalls, and a clear blue lake surrounded by forest, with a relaxing soundtrack. As they were lulled into this serene landscape, cans of Coors Light and Coors Seltzer appeared in the calming scene, disappearing and reappearing several times throughout the clip. People were encouraged to send the link to a friend. If someone tagged a friend @CoorsLight and used #CoorsBigGame Dream on Twitter, they were eligible for a free twelve-pack of Coors Seltzer. After watching the video, people could play an eight-hour relaxing soundscape while they slept.

Malik shared his experience on Instagram live. He woke up around 3 a.m. and described "quite a cool dream." He dreamt of a huge metal robot made of Coors cans that was walking over hills. Malik also dreamt of streams and rivers, reflecting the natural landscape in the Coors clip. "To be honest, I didn't think it was going to work," a sleepy Malik told viewers. "I was quite skeptical. But actually it worked."

My first reaction was a mix of curiosity, suspicion, and uneasiness. This makeshift dream experiment posed a number of philosophical and ethical questions. Was it possible for companies to influence consumers' dreams? If we forget most of our dreams, can advertisements influence our sleeping brain, compelling our waking selves to fill our online cart with products that were peddled to us while we slept? If there was a possibility for companies to guide our dreams, how probable was it?

While we're far from the sci-fi world of *Inception* where a thief broke into people's dreams to steal their secrets, some scientists believe we need to proceed with caution in this brave new world of branded dream content. In 2021, a "Future of Marketing" survey by the American Marketing Association found that 77 percent of four hundred surveyed companies intended to use "dream-tech" advertising by 2025.[13] While this hasn't materialized, there are several companies with multimillion-dollar products that tap into the growing consumer interest in sleep and dreams.

Most notable is Pokémon Sleep, a sleep-tracking game with a unique reward system. At night, a gamer's sleep is tracked using a device's microphone and sensor that detects motion. This includes how long it takes someone to fall asleep and the duration of their sleep. The game categorizes a player's sleep as either dozing, snoozing, or slumbering. The user discovers which Pokémon has the same sleep type, and they receive a sleep score. The higher their "drowsy power," the more Pokémon visit the player. The wildly popular game had 20 million downloads in just over a year and earned $120 million in revenue in its first fourteen months.[14] Countless players have shared their Pokémon dreams online.

In 2020, Microsoft ran its "Made from Dreams" campaign to launch its Series X console. The campaign designed a lucid dreaming experiment in which a recording tried to help participants become lucid and dream about gaming. The Calm app offers "Dune: Caladan" and "Dune: Arrakis" soundscapes based on these two worlds from the movie *Dune*.

Many of us have allowed technology into the private space of our personal lives. Approximately 43 million people in the United States alone have a smart speaker in their home.[15] A recent consumer report found that 45 percent of smart speaker owners have a device in their bedroom.[16] More than one-third of Americans have tried a sleep tracking device, while 77 percent of users found it helpful to use the device.[17] Whether it's for entertainment, self-development, or wellness, many people use digital tools to enhance their personal life, including their sleep and dreams.

I spoke with dream scientists on both sides of the debate over the potential risks of dream advertising. The discussions centred around the issue of consent and the ways in which companies might influence our unconscious thoughts. In the alternate realm of dream advertising, how is informed consent given and what is our capacity for consent when we are fast asleep? Do we know what branded content is being pushed to us while we are out of touch with this world? Could there be a kind of unconscious advertising influence occurring without our knowledge or consent?

Dream studies have shown that at certain times, the dreaming brain is susceptible to suggestion during sleep. Sounds and other stimuli have been used to trigger consolidating of memories, to boost learning, to help dreamers become lucid, and to curb an unwanted habit. With my at-home dream incubation session, I learned how we can guide our thoughts during the first few minutes of sleep. It made me wonder, if dream tech tools are in many of our homes, can companies sell to us while we are asleep and possibly unaware and impressionable?

Several prominent sleep and dream researchers want us to imagine some possible nightmare scenarios. Even though we let sleep trackers collect our data, we might not fully understand how this information is being used, explained Adam Haar, Robert Stickgold, and Antonio Zandra in several opinion pieces on the issue.[18] They posed several scenarios for readers to consider. What if one day companies selling sleep products got access to your sleep data? You might wake up feeling groggy but not realize how bad a night's sleep you really had. Then imagine ads for sleep aids being pushed to you during internet searches. Confectionery companies might take advantage of the connection between sleep loss and sugar, posting ads for whatever candies they are trying to sell.

The researchers referred to a study that found people's candy choice could be swayed if they were exposed to recordings of candy names during Stage 2 of a ninety-minute nap. Subjects had a choice between two familiar candies: M&Ms and Skittles. There wasn't the same effect for subjects who heard the recordings while they were awake.[19]

In one of their articles, the dream researchers pointed to how sleep loss might increase risk-taking behaviours. What if someone with a history of gambling was exposed to an online gambling ad after a restless night? What if the product being promoted was an addictive substance and the message reached those who were struggling with recovery? One study found that crack/cocaine users who dreamt of using a hard drug later experienced a higher degree of craving.[20] I thought of the smokers who smoked less after smelling rotten eggs and cigarettes while they slept. This made me wonder if it was possible to take advantage of suggestion during sleep to encourage an addictive habit.

Who gets to decide what messages are sent to us while we are sleeping and, for the most part, unaware? While an examination of the legal and regulatory aspects of dream advertising is beyond the scope of this book, I learned that subliminal advertising is addressed in certain jurisdictions. In the United States, the Federal Communications Commission (FCC) defines subliminal messaging as "Any technique whereby an attempt is made to convey information to the viewer by transmitting messages below the threshold of normal awareness."[21] Section 5 of the U.S. Federal Trade Commission (FTC) Act prohibits "unfair or deceptive acts or practices in or affecting commerce."[22] Does dream advertising constitute subliminal advertising or deceptive or unfair activities?

Our levels of awareness and cognitive control differ when we are awake compared to when we are asleep. During the day, we use executive thinking and cognitive control to make choices about where our mind goes. Right now, I'm working hard to ignore the beautiful day outside my office window. Yet in a dream, we don't typically have control over events.

Imagine a dream scenario in which I was driving along a road that hugged a cliff, and partway through my dream, I started veering off the narrow, winding road. Even if I wanted to turn the wheel, guiding myself back to safety, my dreaming brain might insist that the frightening scenario play out. I could panic and wake myself up. This would leave the slight chance that if I fell back asleep, I might find myself in a similar situation. (On a couple of rare occasions, I have continued a frightening dream when I dozed off again.)

When we are asleep, our cognitive control is much lower, which could make it easier to guide our thoughts when our defenses are down. "In so many ways, it's such a physically and psychologically vulnerable space," said Haar.

Barrett has studied and practiced dream incubation for several decades. She was asked to consult on the Coors project to share her expertise. She saw it as an opportunity to give people a teaching exercise on dream incubation, even if it had to be oversimplified. Yet Barrett disagreed with the initial "militaristic mind control kind of phrasing" that she felt implied it was involuntary and intrusive. The practice of dream incubation is designed to be voluntary and intentional, with people focusing on a topic that they want to dream about. Also, there wasn't a chance to offer comprehensive dream incubation instructions.

When we talked about dream advertising, Barrett didn't believe that there was an urgent need for new protective policies. While the FTC doesn't specifically address sleep advertising, deceptive or unfair practices apply to all media, even new and emerging ones. Currently, there are only a handful of dream ad campaigns.

Also, Barrett said it would be "a wildly ineffective approach to advertising." She told me that it's just not that powerful to hear messages in your sleep. Things we hear while we sleep, say when we are in REM, can "occasionally get incorporated into your dream without you waking up," Barrett said. "But very occasionally, very subtly, not very powerfully, certainly not overriding what-ever your unconscious is already trying to do in your dream."[23]

In an interview with *Science* magazine, dream researcher Tore Nielsen said his fellow sleep and dream researchers had a "legitimate concern." Yet for such interventions to work, he felt that people needed to be aware of the "manipulation" and be willing to take part in it. Maybe that's why Malik dreamt of Coors cans, because he was open to the experience. Nielsen said he wasn't overly concerned, just as he wasn't worried that people would be hypnotized "against their will."[24]

Lawyer Dustin Marlan offered another perspective on what he called "branding dreams." Dream advertising falls under the parameters of "acts or practices" in Section 5 of the Federal Trade Commission Act, pointed out the assistant professor of law at the University of North Carolina at Chapel

Hill. He looked at the "affecting commerce" language that pertains to anyone involved in commerce, which would include companies doing dream advertising. Marlan pointed to the impact of the Coors project. The dream ad was played 1.4 billion times. Following the ad campaign, there was a 3,000 percent increase in social media engagement and an 8 percent sales increase.[25] By using dream incubation, "branding dreams commodifies the once sacred space of dreams," wrote Marlan.[26]

In 2021, Stickgold, Zadra, and Haar wrote an open letter that received many signatures of support from other researchers in the field. "Our dreams cannot become just another playground for corporate advertisers. Regardless of Coors' intent, their actions set the stage for a corporate assault of our very sense of who we are," wrote the sleep and dream researchers.[27]

The following year, Wunderman Thompson included "dreamvertising" in its annual report on advertising trends to watch that year. While the agency highlighted a growing interest in dream tech among marketers, it suggested that companies approach dream advertising with caution until there was a "deeper scientific understanding."[28] This leaves a lot to think about as you drift off to sleep, possibly with an Amazon Echo or Google Nest by your side.

At the end of my journey through the astonishing and sometimes unsettling new world of dream engineering, I felt cautiously optimistic. If scientists can use technology to influence and guide our dreams, then in theory it is possible to harness this other realm of thought and experience to create big change, both in our waking and dreaming lives. With open and creative dreaming minds, when we are released from waking influences and demands, we could rewrite distressing dreams and cultivate calm, peaceful sleep. We could use our dreams to heal and improve our well-being.

While the initial findings are encouraging, scientists are focused on gathering more observations, more experiments, more evidence. Much as in a dream, we are at the creative brainstorming stage where we chase ideas, stress test theories, and seize the power of possibility. This is just the beginning, and beginnings are full of discovery and promise.

Chapter Thirteen

CONCLUSION: THE INTEROCEPTION OF DREAMS

THERE IS A SCIENTIFIC CONCEPT CALLED INTEROCEPTION, AND it might be the least familiar warning system that resides in each of us. Interoception is our internal sensory system that is sometimes called the eighth sense. Unlike our other senses that recognize what is happening around us, interoception tells us what is happening on the inside.[1] We read our body signals and translate them into feelings. Maybe we realize that we're hungry or thirsty, afraid or in pain.

Here's an example. Imagine that you're walking home at night. You turn off a busy street and realize that you're alone. There's no one in sight. Then you hear the scrape of boots on the sidewalk behind you. You apply information from your senses to create a picture of what's happening.

When you notice the wild thumping of your racing heart against your chest, you experience an uneasiness, and possibly a flicker of panic ignites inside of you. Your interoceptive awareness picks up these internal cues. At less charged moments, you might have overlooked your emotional response to a situation. Sometimes, we are less attuned to the inside story. Maybe we start talking really fast, and when someone says to calm down, we say quite confidently that we aren't excited. We might fail to recognize the signals from our internal sensory system, and our words continue to run together.

One way to understand interoception is to look at the mechanics of the heart. The heart's job is to pump blood, and when it does this, it makes a sound. When the heart beats faster, the sound seems to get louder inside of us. It tells us that something isn't quite right. We are unsettled. In this way, a quickening heartbeat becomes a warning sign calling for our attention. A racing heart might be telling us that we are afraid. Or maybe it signals a mix of nervousness and excitement, like the starting pistol that sets off a race. Whether or not we notice the sound, the heart continues its job of pumping blood. It doesn't beat to make a sound. That isn't what it was designed to do. You can think about dreams in a similar way, suggests sleep and dream expert Robert Stickgold. Dreams do their work, even if we don't remember them.

Dreams strengthen and integrate memories into our lifetime catalogues of experiences and knowledge. Dreams are simulations that help us prepare for risks and uncertainties. The safe space of dreams provides a private therapy session to process difficult emotions and come to terms with the pitfalls and troubles of everyday life. In dreams, we put experiences and their associated emotions into context. We are given different perspectives on ourselves and others while the dreaming brain operates in a different mode. Our dreams can be painfully honest. They illuminate what is weighing on our minds, telling us what remains unsettled.

In the morning, dreams continue to do their work, if we choose to pay attention to them. That's where their use comes in, regardless of their biological function. "The awareness of dreams, when you wake up, is like the heartbeat," explains Stickgold, who founded and served as director of Harvard's Center for Sleep and Cognition for twenty years. Maybe they spark new ideas, which aren't related to the biological construction of a dream. "You know, it can be a freebie," he says.

Dreams exist along our continuum of experience. There is no sharp divide between waking and dreaming life. When we are asleep, our dreams are as real to us as waking experiences. They have the power to influence what we think, feel, and do. Big dreams can transform people's lives, while the quiet, subtle revelations of little dreams seem to bring up what we need. Like the sound of a racing heart, dreams provide information about ourselves. Throughout the night and into the next day, dreams create a kind of mind shift.

During the day, many of us shift our attention and focus inwards as we practice mindfulness and meditation and employ our natural superpower of self-awareness. We might aim to cultivate a growth mindset to rethink what is possible or practice inner reflection in a non-judgmental way to gain insights into ourselves. This is what dreams are designed to do. They act as our brainstormer of ideas and insights. Our creative muse. Our midnight meditation. In dreams, we challenge our beliefs and capabilities.

This idea brought me back to something that dream scientist Adam Haar said when I asked why dreams matter. We can go about our lives without giving dreams a second thought. Why should we pay attention to them? "It's sort of like asking how reflecting on your thoughts or trying to guide your thoughts would benefit you. So kind of a crazy thing to ask," he pointed out. During the day, we apply our waking thoughts to learn, create, and heal. We can do the same with our dreams.

After more than a century of scientific study, researchers continue to investigate many mysteries of the night, including why we construct such complex dream stories. Dreams are random and nonsensical one moment and revelatory the next. Dreams are predictably unpredictable and fixed in their fluidity. In dreams, we are in a constant state of becoming.

Tomorrow morning, take a few extra moments to lie in bed and hold on to your dream before it disappears. It's food for thought. Chew on it for a bit. Turn up your inner awareness and see what your dreams might be telling you. Think about what your dreaming mind created for your benefit, and possibly your curiosity and wonder.

I sit here at my desk, which is strewn with small scraps of paper with random, dreamlike thoughts and ideas to chase. One scribbled note sparks the memory of an otherworldly experience that, in its own way, marks a new beginning for my continued exploration of dreams.

———————

I FIND MYSELF IN a dimly lit room. As my eyes adjust to the darkness, I notice a bed with a large, boxy machine beside it. At first, I think it's an old PSG machine from my dad's first sleep laboratory. I cross the room to take a closer look. There are rows of buttons and switches. I reach for one, then stop myself. With my hand hovering in the air, I notice that I'm all alone. The door is closed. So I grab for one of the switches and the nine-year-old in me flicks it back and forth. Nothing happens. So I do it again. As I hear the satisfying click of the switch, the room flips and becomes my bedroom.

I'm lying in bed, hooked up to the old PSG machine. But instead of monitoring my body and brain activity, it's tracking my dreams. Somehow, I am awake and asleep at the same time. My waking and dreaming worlds have become one. I must be having an exciting dream because the scribbling pens mark page after page until my dream story becomes a tall stack of inked pages, which reminds me of the towers of thousand-page sleep records in my dad's first lab.

I grab the pages from the machine and get back under the covers to read my dream story. It's the best kind of story. A tale of magic realism, with fantastical elements and spellbinding experiences that seem like natural, everyday occurrences. I am with important people in my life, and we are setting out on a quest. I can feel the energy pushing us forward. I don't know where we are going or what we are looking for, but I can't wait to find out. In the corner of my room, there are stacks of dream stories, just waiting to be read. I have created my own private dream lab to study and explore my dreams.

Dreams are their own realm of inner awareness. If I learn to read their signals, just like reading the signals of a racing heart, I may translate their messages into wisdom and wonder. Dreams have the power to illuminate what matters most to us. In dreams, anything is possible. I will take these possibilities with me into tomorrow.

A DREAMER'S TOOLKIT

1. Power Nap

Inspired by Salvador Dalí's "slumber with a key" method and recent scientific findings that show sleep onset is a "creative sweet spot."[1] Use this technique to tap into your natural, sleep-induced brainstormer to find creative ideas.

- With a paper and pen by your side, relax in a comfortable chair.
- Hold a key in one hand. Suspend your arms off the sides of the chair, with the object mid-air above a plate or other hard landing pad.
- Tip your head back and close your eyes.
- Let your mind drift freely.
- As you fall asleep, you will let go of the key. At the sound of the key hitting the plate, quickly write down whatever is on your mind. Enjoy the creative and abstract ideas from your dreamy brainstorming session.

Try This
Don't want to leave your dreams to chance? As you drift off, focus on a specific thought or idea you're working on to discover new insights.

2. Dream Incubation

Dream incubation uses different techniques to help you dream about a chosen topic. Follow these instructions recommended by psychologist and Harvard dream researcher Deirdre Barrett, who has extensively studied dreams and coached people on dream incubation for decades.

- Choose a problem to work on and write it down, placing it by your bed.
- Before you go to bed, review the problem.
- As you lie in bed, visualize the problem as a concrete image, if possible.
- As you drift off, remind yourself that you want to dream about the problem.
- When you wake up, take a few moments to lie quietly in bed. Notice if you can recall any traces of a dream. If so, try and get the dream to return to you.
- Get your paper and pen on your bedside table and write down your dream thoughts.

Bonus Tip

Once you've chosen a problem to work on, you can try to visualize yourself dreaming about the problem, waking up, and writing down what's on your mind. If it's difficult to visualize, place objects beside your bed that are connected to the problem.

3. Lucid Dreaming

Want to try and take control of your dreams? Try these tips on how to lucid dream to gain awareness of the dream state and rescript your dreams as they happen. These suggestions use findings from scientific studies and insights from practiced lucid dreamers.

Reality Checks

- During the day, do reality checks to increase awareness of your waking state, which helps you realize when you are in a dream.
- Check your surroundings to confirm you are awake.
- Examine your hands, which may appear with the wrong number of fingers in dreams.
- Check your reflection in a mirror to see if you look normal.

- Look at a clock to ensure that time is progressing as it should.
- Press your hand against a table or wall, which in a dream can penetrate the hard surface.

Record Your Dreams

When you first wake up, take a few moments to write down your dreams. This makes you pay more attention to dreams and raises awareness of the dream state.

Mnemonic Induction of Lucid Dreams (MILD)

Try this popular lucid dreaming technique by Stephen LaBerge, known as the contemporary father of lucid dreaming. The idea is to visualize yourself in a dream, to realize that you are dreaming, and carry this awareness with you when you return to the dream state.

- Before you fall asleep, tell yourself you will wake up in the night and recall your dreams.
- Wake yourself up during the night. Remember as many details as possible from a dream.
- As you fall back asleep, tell yourself to recognize you are dreaming when you have your next dream. It's not a mantra but rather an intention, like trying to remember your grocery list when shopping.
- When falling asleep, picture yourself in your dream, noticing any "dream signs" that signal it's a dream, like being able to fly or walk through walls.
- As you drift off, remind yourself to recognize you are dreaming when you are in a dream. This helps you enter the dream state with a "meditative focus" and a set goal to become lucid.[2]

How to End a Lucid Dream

If your dream takes a wrong turn and you want to wake up:
- Call for help
- Try to fall asleep in your dream

- Read a book
- Blink

Benefits

Lucid dreaming might help you:
- Rewrite nightmares
- Work on nagging problems
- Experience the impossible
- Master a skill
- Gain psychological insights with the help of a therapist

4. Dream Club

Create your own dream-sharing club to gain new perspectives on your dreams. These instructions follow steps from the popular Montague Ullman dream appreciation method. The psychiatrist believed that people who aren't personally invested in a dream can help us find fresh, unexpected insights to make the most of our nightly stories. Gather a group of fellow dreamers or share your dream with a friend or partner for a quick session in as little as twenty minutes.

- Organize a small group for an online or in-person dream sharing session. The group session may take one hour or longer, depending on discussion.
- Before the session, one person records a dream when it is still fresh in their mind. The person is simply recording all the details they can remember without considering possible interpretations of dream events.
- Someone volunteers to lead the dream-sharing session. The person may be trained in the Ullman method.
- The person who recorded their dream shares it with the group. The person leading the session asks the dreamer to share their remembered feelings, people, places, and dream events.
- Group members ask any necessary clarifying questions about the dream.

- The group is asked to imagine thoughts and feelings if it was their dream to provide a diversity of perspectives. The Ullman method has people fill in the sentence, "If it were my dream . . ." The dreamer discovers the elements that would have resonated with others if it was their dream.
- The dreamer can address people's comments or keep their thoughts to themselves for personal reflection later on.
- The dreamer shares what was happening in their waking life leading up to the dream, paying close attention to what was on their mind the day and evening before the dream. This includes any preoccupations, concerns, or possibly conversations that continue to occupy their thoughts.
- A group member, possibly the person leading the session, reads the dream back to the dreamer in the second person to offer another perspective. The dreamer can add any details that now come to mind about the dream or waking events leading up to the dream.
- The group works together to find any connections between the dreamer's waking and dreaming lives. This includes metaphorical and literal connections between what was happening in the person's waking life and people, emotions, or events reflected in their dream.
- The dreamer is given new insights and ways of seeing their dream, which they can continue to reflect on and appreciate.

Bonus Tip:

To record more details, sensations, and emotions of your dreams, make a voice recording as you lay in bed with your eyes closed and the dream is still fresh in your mind. Then transcribe the recording and share it with your dream club.

5. Fight Dream Deprivation

A recent study found we're as dream deprived as we are sleep deprived as we cut our nights short and rob ourselves of REM sleep.[3] Try these healthy habits, see which ones work for you, and create your own sleep system.

Habits for Healthy Sleep

- During the day, exercise and get outside to regulate circadian rhythms and sleep patterns.
- Create a dark, cool, and quiet environment for sleep.
- Maintain a regular sleep schedule, falling asleep and waking around the same time each day.
- Limit alcohol, which can cause a bad night's sleep with reduced REM and frequent awakenings.
- Avoid caffeine or exercise later in the day.
- Enjoy the comforts of a bedtime routine. Avoid screens before bed and do something relaxing that you learn to associate with sleep.

6. Cultivate Calm Sleep

Lying in bed ruminating over negative thoughts can make it difficult to drift off or have a good night's sleep. A recent study found that how we think about someone who's offended us helps with "emotional repair," increases forgiveness, and may lead to a better night's sleep. Try these compassionate reappraisal techniques from psychology professor Charlotte vanOyen-Witvliet to practice positivity and quiet negative ruminations.[4] The key to a good night's sleep might be finding forgiveness for the person who's hurt you.

- Recognize the humanity of the person who's offended you. Understand, don't excuse, where they are coming from.
- Acknowledge how you've been wronged and the impact it's made. Don't minimize your hurt.
- Take another look at what's been done to you. Reconsider it as evidence that the person needs positive change.
- Genuinely wish that the person who's hurt you experiences good change, even if you can't repair your relationship.

7. Dream Collector

Keeping a regular dream diary can improve dream recall, letting you build a collection of dreams to reflect on. Analyzing a series of dreams helps identify recurring elements and themes that you can connect with what's happening in your waking life or compare to other people's dreams. All you need is a paper and pen and some motivation to make it part of your routine.

- Keep your dream journal by your bedside.
- When you wake up, spend a few moments lying in bed, thinking about your dreams.
- Quickly write down your thoughts before they disappear.
- Connect your dreams with what's happening in your waking life. See if themes pop up at certain times.
- Compare common elements or emotions to those in other people's dreams using the tools below.

Tools

The Hall/Van de Castle coding system is a popular dream analysis tool. It also has a set of norms to compare frequency of dream elements. For excellent instructions on content analysis, see G. William Domhoff's "Coding Rules for the Hall/Van de Castle System of Quantitative Dream Content Analysis" at https://dreams.ucsc.edu/Coding/.

Sleep and Dream Database (SDDB) is a searchable digital collection of more than forty thousand dreams. See how political ideology relates to visitation dreams, compare dream recall by gender, or customize your own dream analysis at https://sleepanddreamdatabase.org/.

DreamBank.net is a free online database of more than twenty thousand dream reports. Use the database to conduct your own dream analysis. Compare the frequency of elements in your dreams to anonymized dream reports to see how common or rare they are.

Elsewhere is one of many digital analysis tools. The dream journal app tracks dreams across time so you can connect your waking and dreaming lives. It offers insights on recurring elements and art generation of your dreams. Try its different interpretation modes, including Freudian and Jungian analyses.

The **Dust** app has several programs to make the most of your dreams. Learn ways to improve your dream recall, guide your dreams, and reduce nightmares.

ACKNOWLEDGEMENTS

IN OUR SLEEP-DEPRIVED SOCIETY, IT CAN SEEM NEXT TO IMPOS-sible to think about our dreams when we're struggling to get a good night's sleep. I've discovered how nourishing ourselves with dream sleep and tuning into our dreams can improve and enrich our waking lives. To my dad, Murray Moffat, thank you for opening my eyes to the world of sleep, the gateway to the fascinating realm of dreams. To my mom, Linda Moffat, thank you for passing on your curiosity to keep learning and your love of reading. To Dimitri van Kampen, my first reader and partner in life, thank you for the inspiring brainstorming sessions, for pushing me to keep writing, and for going along with a dream experiment. To my kind, thoughtful kids, Alexander and Claudia, thank you for your support, and for patiently listening to my excited ramblings about the dreaming brain.

To my fabulous literary agent, Amy Tompkins, thank you for your guidance and support and for finding a home for "the dream book." To my amazing speaker agent, Rob Firing, thank you for helping me spread the word about dreams. Thank you to Samantha Haywood and the incredible team at Transatlantic Agency for your ongoing support. To Jim Gifford, my exceptional book editor, thank you for your keen eye, editorial insights, and thoughtful perspectives that guided my manuscript. I'm so fortunate to work with you again. To the wonderful team at Simon & Schuster Canada, including Paul Barker, Muna Hussein, Phil Metcalf, Maya Price-Baker, Carine Redmond, and Lisa Wray, thank you for supporting this book and for all that you do. I'm thrilled to be one of your authors.

To all the dream researchers, scientists, doctors, patients, and passionate dreamers, thank you for sharing your time and dizzying knowledge on the confounding world of dreams, and for your guidance in helping me deconstruct dream science. For the many lengthy conversations, thanks to Armond Aserinsky, Benjamin Baird, Thomas J. Balkin, Deirdre Barrett, Allen R. Braun, the late Roger Broughton, Kelly Bulkeley, Harrison Chow, Andrew Gall, Laura Hack, the late Ernest Hartmann, Keith Hearne, Boris Heifets, the late J. Allan Hobson, Karen Konkoly, Megan Kozak Williams, Susan Chana Lask, Julia Lockheart, Mare Lucas, the late Mark Mahowald, Janet Makinen, Michael Mangan, Christopher Mazurek, Jay McClelland, Patrick McNamara, David Neubauer, Kelsey Newman, Ken Paller, Antti Revonsuo, David R. Samson, Michael Schredl, Colin Shapiro, Pilleriin Sikka, Carlyle Smith, Elizaveta Solomonova, Mark Solms, Neil Stanley, Philippe Stenstrom, Charlotte vanOyen-Witvliet, the late Daniel M. Wegner, and Antonio Zadra. I will never look at my dreams the same way again.

A special thanks to Mark Blagrove and Julia Lockheart for hosting an online dream salon. Thank you, Julia, for my canvas of dreams that is hanging beside me at my desk, reminding me of the special experience. To my dream sharing group that joined from across Canada, the United States, and the UK, thank you for spending a wintery Saturday morning sharing your perspectives and insights into my dreams. This includes Subo Awan, Ali Awan, Deirdre Barrett, Lisa Beaudoin, Deirdre Daly, Tony Discenza, Ivana Marzura, Margot Perlmutter, and Paul Stocks.

To Robert Stickgold, thank you for the many fascinating conversations on dreams and memory and for the visit to the Beth Israel Deaconess Medical Center of Harvard Medical School, where I tested out my own version of the downhill skiing dream experiment.

To Tore Nielsen and the team at the Dream and Nightmare Laboratory in Montreal, thank you for the overnight visit so I could better understand what dreams are made of.

To Adam Haar, thanks for helping me set up my own at-home dream experiment so I could experience the possibilities of guiding my dreams. Thank you all for opening up my world of dreams.

Notes

1. "Freud, Dalí and the Metamorphosis of Narcissus," Freud Museum London, accessed November 24, 2024, https://www.freud.org.uk/exhibitions/freud-dali-and-the-metamorphosis-of-narcissus/.
2. Salvador Dalí, *Conquest of the Irrational*, trans. David Gascoyne (New York: Julien Levy, 1935), 12. For background, also see D. A. Gordon, "Experimental Psychology and Modern Painting," *Journal of Aesthetics and Art Criticism* 9, no. 2, (March 1951): 227–243, and "Paranoid-Critical Method," Tufts University, accessed November 24, 2024, https://mma.pages.tufts.edu/fah188/clifford/Subsections/Paranoidpercent20Critical/paranoidcriticalmethod.html#:~:text=Afterpercent20hispercent20selfpercent2Dinducedpercent20paranoid,opticalpercent20illusionspercent20andpercent20juxtaposing percent20images.
3. Salvador Dalí, *50 Secrets of Magic Craftsmanship* (New York: Dover, 1992), 36. Originally published 1948.
4. Célia Lacaux et al., "Sleep Onset Is a Creative Sweet Spot," *Science Advances* 7, no. 50 (December 10, 2021): eabj5866, doi.org/10.1126/sciadv.abj5866.
5. Rubin Naiman, "Dreamless: The Silent Epidemic of REM Sleep Loss," *Annals of the New York Academy of Sciences* 1406, no. 1 (October 2017): 77–85.

Chapter One: The Freud Effect

1. Sigmund Freud, *The Diary of Sigmund Freud 1929–1939: A Record of the Final Decade*, trans. Michael Molnar (London: The Hogarth Press, 1992), 248.
2. Sigmund Freud, *The Interpretation of Dreams*, trans. Joyce Crick (Oxford: Oxford University Press, 1999), 86.
3. Calvin Kai-Ching Yu, "Dream Motif Scale," *Dreaming* 22, no. 1 (November 2011): 18–52, doi: 10.1037/a0026171.
4. Naama Rozen and Nirit Soffer-Dudek, "Dreams of Teeth Falling Out: An Empirical Investigation of Physiological and Psychological Correlates," *Frontiers in Psychology* 9 (September 25, 2018): 1–8, doi.org/10.3389/fpsyg.2018.01812.
5. Freud, *Diary of Sigmund Freud 1929–1939*, 247.
6. Background on Freud, including the thread of his unconscious woven through his antiquities collection, from interview with Michael Molnar, former director of the Freud Museum in London.
7. Freud, *Interpretation of Dreams*, x–xi.

8. W. B. Webb, "Retrospective Review: Sigmund Freud's The Interpretation of Dreams," *Dreaming* 4, no. 1 (1994): 56.

9. Alfred Maury, *Le Sommeil et les Rêves* (Paris: Didier, 1865), 1–2.

10. Ian Dowbiggin, "Alfred Maury and the Politics of the Unconscious in Nineteenth-Century France," *History Of Psychiatry* 1, no. 3 (1990): 283, https://doi.org/10.1177/09571 54X9000100301.

11. Dowbiggin, "Alfred Maury": 284.

12. For excellent background on pioneering dream researchers, see Antonio Zadra and Robert Stickgold, *When Brains Dream: Understanding the Science and Mystery of Our Dreaming Minds* (New York: W. W. Norton & Company, 2021).

13. Hervey de Saint-Denys, *Les Rêves et les Moyens De Les Diriger: Observations Pratiques* (Dreams and the Ways to Direct Them: Practical Observations), ebook, eds. Carolus den Blanken and Eli Meijer, 2016 (Paris: Amyot, 1867), 7.

14. Saint-Denys, *Les Rêves*, 8. For background on Alfred Maury and Hervey de Saint-Denys's work, see Tony James, *Dream, Creativity, and Madness in Nineteenth-Century France* (Oxford: Oxford University Press, 1995), 169–183.

15. Saint-Denys, *Les Rêves*, 17.

16. Saint-Denys, *Les Rêves*, 18.

17. Saint-Denys, *Les Rêves*, 157.

18. Saint-Denys, *Les Rêves*, 159.

19. Saint-Denys, *Les Rêves*, 120.

20. Saint-Denys, *Les Rêves*, 120.

21. Mary Whiton Calkins, " Statistics of Dreams," *American Journal of Psychology* 5, no. 3 (April 1893): 312. Note: footnote states "experimenter," which could refer to Calkins or Sanford.

22. Calkins, " Statistics of Dreams": 315.

23. Mary Whiton Calkins, "Autobiography of Mary Whiton Calkins," *History of Psychology in Autobiography* 1 (1930): 31–61. Republished by the permission of Clark University Press, Worcester, MA. https://psychclassics.yorku.ca/Calkins/murchison.htm.

24. Calkins, " Statistics of Dreams": 320.

25. Calkins, "Autobiography": 31–61.

26. Calkins, "Autobiography": 31–61.

27. C. W. O'Nell, *Dreams, Culture and the Individual* (San Francisco: Chandler and Sharp Publishers Inc., 1976), 32.

28. O'Nell, *Dreams, Culture and the Individual*, 32.

Chapter Two: The Peaks and Valleys of Sleep

1. Background of Eugene Aserinsky's life and work from interviews with his son, Armond Aserinsky.

2. Lynne Lamberg, "The Student, the Professor and the Birth of Modern Sleep Research," *Medicine on the Midway* (Spring 2004): 18.

3. William Dement and Christopher Vaughan, *The Promise of Sleep: A Pioneer in Sleep Medicine Explores the Vital Connection Between Health, Happiness, and a Good Night's Sleep* (New York: Delacorte Press, 1999), 35.

4. Dement and Vaughan, *Promise of Sleep*, 40.

5. Background on the late J. Allan Hobson's life and work from interviews with subject.

6. Background on Michel Jouvet's work, see Mark Solms and Oliver Turnbull, *The Brain and the Inner World: An Introduction to the Neuroscience of Subjective Experience* (New York: Other Press, 2002), 185–186; J. Allan Hobson, *The Dreaming Brain: How the Brain Creates Both the Sense and the Nonsense of Dreams* (New York: Basic Books, 1988).

7. J. Allan Hobson and Robert W. McCarley, "The Brain as Dream State Generator: An Activation Synthesis Hypothesis of the Dream Process," *American Journal of Psychiatry* 134, no. 12 (December 1977): 1347.

8. Hobson and McCarley, "The Brain as Dream State Generator": 1346.

9. W. D. Foulkes, "Dream Reports from Different Stages of Sleep," *Journal of Abnormal and Social Psychology* 65, no. 1 (1962): 14–25, https://doi.org/10.1037/h0040431.

10. Oliver Sacks, *A Leg to Stand On* (London: Duckworth, 1984), 164.

11. Background on Mark Solms's life and work, from interviews with subject. Also see Mark Solms, "Dreaming and REM Sleep Are Controlled by Different Brain Mechanisms," *Behavioral and Brain Sciences* 23 (2000): 846.

12. J. Allan Hobson, Charles C.-H. Hong, and Karl J. Friston, "Virtual Reality and Consciousness Inference in Dreaming," *Front. Psychol.* 5, no. 1133 (October 2014): 1–18.

13. Kieran C.R. Fox et al., "Dreaming as Mind Wandering: Evidence From Functional Neuroimaging and First-person Content Reports," *Front Hum Neurosci.* 7 (July 30, 2013): 412, doi: 10.3389/fnhum.2013.00412. PMID: 23908622; PMCID: PMC3726865; and G. William Domhoff and Kieran C.R. Fox, "Dreaming and the Default Network: A Review, Synthesis, and Counterintuitive Research Proposal," *Conscious Cogn.* 33 (May 2015): 342-53, doi: 10.1016/j.concog.2015.01.019. Epub 2015 Feb 24. PMID: 25723600.

Chapter Three: The Dark Side of the Dreaming Mind

1. Court of Appeal for Ontario. Her Majesty the Queen and Jan Luedecke. Respondent's Factum. (January 22, 2008): 2.

2. Court of Appeal for Ontario. Respondent's Factum: 5.

3. Court of Appeal for Ontario. Respondent's Factum: 3.

4. American Academy of Sleep Medicine, "REM Sleep Behavior Disorder as a Prodrome of Neurodegenerative Disorders," Provider Fact Sheet, https://aasm.org/wp-content/uploads/2022/07/ProviderFS-REM-Sleep-Behavior-Disorder.pdf (accessed March 25, 2025). For statistics on general population and older adults, see Imran Khawaja, Benjamin C. Spurling, and Shantanu Singh, "REM Sleep Behavior Disorder," *StatPearls* (StatPearls Publishing, 2023), 3.

5. For background and statistics on nightmares, see Michael Schredl, *Researching Dreams: The Fundamentals* (Switzerland: Palgrave Macmillan, 2018).

6. Stephanie Saul, "Study Links Ambien Use to Unconscious Food Forays," *New York Times*, March 14, 2006, https://www.nytimes.com/2006/03/14/health/study-links-ambien-use -to-unconscious-food-forays.html.

7. Background on civil suit and Susan Chana Lask's work, from interviews with subject.

8. "FDA Requests Label Change for All Sleep Disorder Drug Products," FDA News, March 14, 2007.

9. C. H. Schenck, "Update on Sexsomnia, Sleep Related Sexual Seizures, and Forensic Implications," *NeuroQuant* 13 (2015): 518–541.

10. B. J. Holoyda et al., "Forensic Evaluation of Sexsomnia," *Journal of the American Academy of Psychiatry and Law* 49, no. 2 (June 2021): 202–210, doi: 10.29158/JAAPL.200077-20, epub 2021 Feb 12, PMID: 33579735.

11. Court of Appeal for Ontario. Respondent's Factum: 6.

12. Court of Appeal for Ontario. Respondent's Factum: 12.

13. This is a Canadian interpretation of the law. In the UK, the M'Naghten Rule is a legal test used as a basis to determine criminal insanity. For further reading on non-insane automatism, see the leading Canadian case *R v. Stone* [1999], 2 S.C.R. 290. Also see *R v. Fontaine* [2004], 183 C.C. C. (3d) 1 (S.C.C.).

14. Description of Parks case and quotation from *R. v. Parks*. O.J. 880 Ontario Court of Appeal, June 1, 1990.

15. For quotation and following quotation from Roger Broughton, see *R. v. Parks* O.J. 880 Ontario Court of Appeal, June 1, 1990.

16. *R. v. Luedecke*, 2005 ONCJ 294, p. 14. For more background on case, see *R. v. Parks* S.C.J. 71, January 27, 1992.

Chapter Four: Dreams and Our Mental Health

1. Several studies showed the impact of COVID-19 on our dreams, including M. Gorgoni et al., "Pandemic Dreams: Quantitative and Qualitative Features of the Oneric Activity During the Lockdown Due to COVID-19 in Italy," *Sleep Medicine* 81 (May 2021): 20–32, doi: 10.1016/j.sleep.2021.02.006.

2. For an excellent explanation of how COVID changed our dreams, see T. Nielsen, "The COVID-19 Pandemic Is Changing Our Dreams," *Scientific American*, October 1, 2020, https://www.scientificamerican.com/article/the-covid-19-pandemic-is-changing-our -dreams/. For background on how COVID impacted our sleep quantity and quality, see C. Blume et al., "Effects of the COVID-19 Lockdown on Human Sleep and Rest-Activity Rhythms," *Current Biology* 30, no. 4 (July 20, 2020): R795–R797.

3. I. Sample, "Covid Poses 'Greatest Threat to Mental Health Since Second World War,'" *Guardian*, December 27, 2020, https://www.theguardian.com/society/2020/dec/27/covid -poses-greatest-threat-to-mental-health-since-second-world-war.

4. For background on how COVID-19 impacted our mental health and the bidirectional relationship between dreams and mental health, see E. Solomonova, "Stuck in a Lockdown: Dreams, Bad Dreams, Nightmares, and Their Relationship to Stress, Depression and Anxiety During the COVID-19 Pandemic," *PLoS One* 16, no. 11 (November 24, 2021): e0259040, doi: 10.1371/journal.pone.0259040.eCollection 2021.

5. C. Franceschini et al., "Poor Sleep Quality and Its Consequences on Mental Health During the COVID-19 Lockdown in Italy," *Frontiers in Psychology* 11 (November 9, 2020): 574475, doi: 10.3389/fpsyg.2020.574475, PMID: 33304294, PMCID: PMC7693628.

6. Among the studies on the bidirectional relationship between sleep and stress is Y Yap et al., "Bi-directional Relations Between Stress and Self-Reported and Actigraphy-Assessed Sleep: A Daily Intensive Longitudinal Study," *Sleep* 43, no. 3 (March 12, 2020): zsz250, doi: 10.1093/sleep/zsz250, PMID: 31608395, PMCID: PMC7066487.

7. M. Schredl and K. Bulkeley, "Dreaming and the COVID-19 Pandemic: A Survey in a U.S. Sample," *Dreaming* 30, no. 3 (2020): 189–198, https://doi.org/10.1037/drm0000146.

8. Nielsen, "COVID-19 Pandemic Is Changing Our Dreams."

9. For background on idreamofcovid.com and descriptions of dream patterns, see "'I Dream of Covid' Tracks Subconscious Under Quarantine," *All Things Considered* on NPR, April 13, 2020, https://www.npr.org/2020/04/13/833623332/i-dream-of-covid-tracks-subconscious-under-quarantine; T. Worley, "The Plant Scientist Who's Analyzing People's Pandemic Dreams," Ideo, May 2020, https://www.ideo.com/journal/the-plant-scientist-whos-analyzing-peoples-pandemic-dreams.

10. For background and study results, see M. Schredl and K. Bulkeley, "Dreaming and the COVID-19 Pandemic: A Survey in a U.S. Sample," *Dreaming* 30, no. 3 (2020): 189–198, https://doi.org/10.1037/drm0000146.

11. For background on Deirdre Barrett's work and her findings on dreams during the COVID-19 pandemic, see Deirdre Barrett, *Pandemic Dreams* (Oneiroi Press, 2020), Kindle.

12. Barrett, *Pandemic Dreams*, 53.

13. Barrett, *Pandemic Dreams*, 37.

14. Ibid, 36.

15. S. Scarpelli et al., "Pandemic Nightmares: Effects on Dream Activity of the COVID-19 Lockdown in Italy," *Journal of Sleep Research* 30, no. 5 (October 2021): e13300, doi: 10.1111/jsr.13300.

16. Solomonova, "Stuck in a Lockdown."

17. Description of dream and background on Zadra's work from conversation with Antonio Zadra. Also see A. Zadra, "Understanding Lucid Dreaming," TEDxMarinSalon, April 2021, https://www.ted.com/talks/antonio_zadra_understanding_lucid_dreaming?subtitle=en.

18. For background on recurrent dreams and their connection with well-being, see R. J. Brown and D. C. Donderi, "Dream Content and Self-Reported Well-Being Among Recurrent Dreamers, Past-Recurrent Dreamers, and Nonrecurrent Dreamers," *Journal of Personality and Social Psychology* 50, no. 3 (1986): 612–623, https://doi.org/10.1037/0022-3514.50.3.612.

19. A. Zadra et al., "Evolutionary Function of Dreams: A Test of the Threat Simulation Theory in Recurrent Dreams," *Conscious Cogn* 15, no. 2 (June 2006): 450–63, doi: 10.1016/j.con cog.2005.02.002. For background on recurrent dreams, see A. Zadra, "Recurrent Dreams: Their Relation to Life Events," in *Trauma and Dreams*, ed. Deirdre Barrett (Harvard University Press, 1996), 231–248.

20. A. Rimsh and R. Pietrowsky,"Analysis of Dream Contents of Patients with Anxiety Disorders and Their Comparison with Dreams of Healthy Participants," *Dreaming* 31, no. 4 (2021): 303–319, https://doi.org/10.1037/drm0000184.

21. For background on Carl Jung's house dream and Jungian dream interpretation, see Kelly Bulkeley, *An Introduction to the Psychology of Dreaming* (Westport, CT: Praeger, 1997), 33–34.

22. R. D. Cartwright, "The Nature and Function of Repetitive Dreams: A Speculation," *Psychiatry* 42 (1979): 131–137.

23. For background on study and Carl Jung's views of recurrent dreams, see Brown and Donderi, "Dream Content."

24. N. Pesant and A. Zadra, "Dream Content and Psychological Well-Being: A Longitudinal Study of the Continuity Hypothesis," *Journal of Clinical Psychology* 62, no. 1 (January 2006): 111–121, doi: 10.1002/jclp.20212, PMID: 16288448.

25. For background on well-being and dreams and findings on peace of mind and dreaming, see P. Sikka et al., "Peace of Mind and Anxiety in the Waking State are Related to the Affective Content of Dreams," *Scientific Reports* 8, no. 1 (August 24, 2018): 12762, https://doi.org/10.1038 /s41598-018-30721-1.

26. National Sleep Foundation, "2012 Sleep in America Poll—Transportation Workers' Sleep," *Sleep Health* 1, no. 2 (June 2015): e11, doi: 10.1016/j.sleh.2015.04.011; also see R. E. Schmidt et al., "Too Imperfect to Fall Asleep: Perfectionism, Pre-sleep Counterfactual Processing, and Insomnia," *Frontiers of Psychology* 9 (August 7, 2018): 1288, doi: 10.3389 /fpsyg.2018.01288, PMID: 30131735, PMCID: PMC6090461.

27. X. Feng X and J. Wang, "Presleep Ruminating on Intrusive Thoughts Increased the Possibility of Dreaming of Threatening Events," *Frontiers of Psychology* 13 (January 26, 2022): 809131, doi: 10.3389/fpsyg.2022.809131.

28. For description of nightmare content, see Geneviéve Robert and Antonio Zadra, "Thematic and Content Analysis of Idiopathic Nightmares and Bad Dreams," *Sleep* 37, no. 2 (February 1, 2014): 409-17, doi: 10.5665/sleep.3426.

29. For background and statistics on nightmares, see M. Schredl, *Researching Dreams: The Fundamentals* (Switzerland: Palgrave Macmillan, 2018).

30. T. Nielsen, "The Stress Acceleration Hypothesis of Nightmares," *Frontiers in Neurology* 8 (June 1, 2017): 201, https://doi.org/10.3389/fneur.2017.00201.

31. Schredl, *Researching Dreams.*

32 N. Sandman et al, "Nightmares as Predictors of Suicide: An Extension Study Including War Veterans," *Scientific Reports* 7 (March 15, 2017): 44756, https://doi.org/10.1038 /srep44756.

33. M. El-Hourani et al., "Longitudinal Associations Throughout Adolescence: Suicidal Ideation, Disturbing Dreams, and Internalizing Symptoms," *Sleep Medicine* 98 (October 2022): 89–97, https://doi.org/10.1016/j.sleep.2022.06.012.

34. For background on disturbing dreams and suicide among adolescents, see A. Gauchat et al., "Association Between Recurrent Dreams, Disturbing Dreams, and Suicidal Ideation in Adolescents," *Dreaming* 31, no. 1 (2021): 32–43, https://doi.org/10.1037/drm0000157.

35. For statistics and background on nightmares, see Schredl, *Researching Dreams.*

36. For statistics on nightmare support, see Schredl, *Researching Dreams.*

37. Westley Youngren et al., "Exploring Dream Self-Efficacy's Relationship with Suicide," *Sleep*, 48, issue supplement 1 (May 19, 2025): A516, https://doi.org/10.1093/sleep/zsaf090.1195.

38. D. M. Wegner et al., "Dream Rebound: The Return of Suppressed Thoughts in Dreams," *Psychological Science* 15, no. 4 (April 2004): 232–236, https://doi.org/10.1111/j.0963-7214.2004.00657.x.

39. L. Winerman, "Suppressing the 'White Bears,'" *Monitor on Psychology* 42, no. 9 (October 2011), https://www.apa.org/monitor/2011/10/unwanted-thoughts.

Chapter Five: The Safe Space of Dreams

1. Background on Cartwright's lab, studies and career, see K. Tingley, "Rosalind Cartwright," *New York Times Magazine*, December 26, 2021, https://www.nytimes.com/interactive/2021/12/22/magazine/rosalind-cartwright-death.html; P. Green, "Rosalind Cartwright, Psychologist and 'Queen of Dreams,' Dies at 98," *New York Times*, March 15, 2021, https://www.nytimes.com/2021/03/15/obituaries/rosalind-cartwright-dead.html.

2. P. Green, "Rosalind Cartwright."

3. For quotations, reflections on Cartwright's personal life, and background on her career, see R. Cartwright and L. Lamberg, *Crisis Dreaming: Using Your Dreams to Solve Your Problems* (San Jose: ASJA Press, 2000), 6, originally published 1992 by HarperCollins.

4. Cartwright and Lamberg, *Crisis Dreaming*, 12.

5. For background on Hartmann's central image concept, dreaming's connection to psychotherapy, and his theory on the boundaries in the mind, see Ernest Hartmann, *Boundaries in the Mind: A New Psychology of Personality* (New York: Basic Books, 1991); Ernest Hartmann, *Dreams and Nightmares: The Origin and Meaning of Dreams* (Cambridge: Perseus Publishing, 1998); E. Hartmann, "Outline for a Theory on the Nature and Functions of Dreaming," *Dreaming* 6, no. 2 (1996): 147–170.

6. Information on the impact of 9/11 on dreams, from interview with subject; also see E. Hartmann and T. Brezler, "A Systematic Change in Dreams After 9/11/01," *Sleep* 31, no. 2 (February 1, 2008): 213–218; E. Hartmann and R. Basile, "Dream Imagery Becomes More Intense After 9/11," *Dreaming* 13, no. 2 (June 2003): 213–218.

7. Description of study and results of Boundary Questionnaire, see Ernest Hartmann, *Boundaries in the Mind,* 146–155.

8. From interviews with subject.

9. For background on emotional processing and regulation in sleep and dreams, see M. Vandekerckhove and Y. L. Wang, "Emotion, Emotion Regulation and Sleep: An Intimate Relationship," *AIMS Neuroscience* 5, no. 1 (December 1, 2017): 1–17, https://doi.org/10.3934/Neuroscience.2018.1.1.

10. Vandekerckhove and Wang, "Emotion, Emotion Regulation and Sleep."

11. Quotations from Mattew Walker, see Matthew Walker, *Why We Sleep: Unlocking the Power of Sleep and Dreams* (New York: Scribner, 2017), 208–209. For background on emotional processing in dreams including brain activity, see S. Scarpelli et al., "The Functional Role of Dreaming in Emotional Processes," *Frontiers in Psychology* 10 (March 15, 2019): 459, https://doi.org/10.3389/fpsyg.2019.00459; Matthew P. Walker, "The Role of Sleep in Cognition and Emotion," *Annals of the New York Academy of Sciences* 1156 (March 2009): 168–197, https://doi.org/10.1111/j.1749-6632.2009.04416.x.

12. Els van der Helm and Matthew P. Walker, "Overnight Therapy? The Role of Sleep in Emotional Brain Processing," *Psychological Bulletin* 135, no. 5 (September 2009): 731–748, https://doi.org/10.1037/a0016570. For excellent background on the model of dreaming as overnight therapy, see Walker, *Why We Sleep,* 206–218.

13. Walker, *Why We Sleep,* 210.

14. For dream reports and background on the study, see D. R. Samson et al., "Evidence for an Emotional Adaptive Function of Dreams: A Cross-Cultural Study," *Scientific Reports* 13, no. 1 (October 2, 2023): 16530, https://doi.org/10.1038/s41598-023-43319-z.

15. D. Foulkes, *Dreaming: A Cognitive-Psychological Analysis* (Hillsdale, NJ: Lawrence Erlbaum, 1985).

16. A. Revonsuo, "The Reinterpretation of Dreams: An Evolutionary Hypothesis of the Function of Dreaming," *Behavioral and Brain Sciences* 23, no. 6 (December 2000): 877–901, https://doi.org/10.1017/s0140525x00004015.

17. Katja Valli et al., "The Threat Simulation Theory of the Evolutionary Function of Dreaming: Evidence from Dreams of Traumatized Children," *Consciousness and Cognition* 14, no. 1 (2005): 188–218.

18. Isabelle Arnulf et al., "Will Students Pass a Competitive Exam That They Failed in Their Dreams?" *Consciousness and Cognition* 29 (October 2014): 43, https://doi.org/10.1016/j.concog.2014.06.010.

19. Isabelle Arnulf et al., "Will Students Pass a Competitive Exam," 46.

20. V. Sterpenich et al., "Fear in Dreams and in Wakefulness: Evidence for Day/Night Affective Homeostasis," *Human Brain Mapping* 41, no. 3 (February 15, 2020): 840–850, https://doi.org/10.1002/hbm.24843.

21. Antti Revonsuo and Jarno Tuominen, "Avatars in the Machine: Dreaming as a Simulation of Social Reality," *Open MIND* (2015): 28, https://doi.org/10.15502/9783958570375.

Chapter Six: What Dreams Are Made Of

1. M. J. Fosse et al., "Dreaming and Episodic Memory: A Functional Dissociation?," *Journal of Cognitive Neuroscience* 15, no. 1 (January 1, 2003): 1–9, https://doi.org/10.1162/089892 903321107774.
2. C. Picard-Deland et al., "The Memory Sources of Dreams: Serial Awakenings Across Sleep Stages and Time of Night," *Sleep* 46, no. 4 (April 12, 2023): zsac292, https://doi .org/10.1093/sleep/zsac292.
3. Information on Dream Lag Effect from interviews with Tore Nielsen; also see Tore A. Nielsen et al., "Immediate and Delayed Incorporations of Events into Dreams: Further Replication and Implications for Dream Function," *Journal of Sleep Research* 13, no. 4 (December 2004): 327–336, https://doi.org/10.1111/j.1365-2869.2004.00421.x.

Chapter Seven: Making Memories Stick

1. U. Neisser and N. Harsch, "Phantom Flashbulbs: False Recollections of Hearing the News About Challenger," in *Affect and Accuracy in Recall: Studies of 'Flashbulb' Memories*, ed. E. Winograd and U. Neisser (Cambridge: Cambridge University Press, 1992), 9–31, https:// doi.org/10.1017/CBO9780511664069.003.
2. Fiona Gabbert et al., "Memory Conformity Between Eyewitnesses," *Court Review: The Journal of the American Judges Association* (2012): 382, https://digitalcommons.unl.edu /ajacourtreview/382. For the next cited study by Gabbert and colleagues, see Fiona Gabbert, Amina Memon, and Kevin Allan, "Memory Conformity: Can Eyewitnesses Influence Each Other's Memories for an Event?," *Applied Cognitive Psychology* 17, no. 5 (July 2003): 533–543.
3. Els van der Helm and Matthew P. Walker, "Overnight Therapy? The Role of Sleep in Emotional Brain Processing," *Psychological Bulletin* 135, no. 5 (September 2009): 731–748, https://doi.org/10.1037/a0016570. For excellent background on the model of dreaming as overnight therapy, see Matthew Walker, *Why We Sleep: Unlocking the Power of Sleep and Dreams* (New York: Scribner, 2017).
4. William James, *Principles of Psychology* (New York: Holt, 1890), 670.
5. S. O. Yoon, M. C. Duff, and S. Brown-Schmidt, "Learning and Using Knowledge About What Other People Do and Don't Know Despite Amnesia," *Cortex* 94 (September 2017): 164–175, https://doi.org/10.1016/j.cortex.2017.06.020.
6. Details of the Tetris study from conversations with Robert Stickgold; also see Robert Stickgold et al., "Replaying the Game: Hypnagogic Images in Normals and Amnesiacs," *Science* 290 (October 13, 2000): 350–353.
7. E. J. Wamsley et al., "Cognitive Replay of Visuomotor Learning at Sleep Onset: Temporal Dynamics and Relationship to Task Performance," *Sleep* 33, no. 1 (January 2010): 59–68, https://doi.org/10.1093/sleep/33.1.59.

8. B. Rasch et al., "Odor Cues During Slow-Wave Sleep Prompt Declarative Memory Consolidation," *Science* 315, no. 5817 (March 9, 2007): 1426–1429, https://doi.org/10.1126/science.1138581.

9. J. D. Rudoy et al., "Strengthening Individual Memories by Reactivating Them During Sleep," *Science* 326, no. 5956 (November 20, 2009): 1079, https://doi.org/10.1126/science.1179013.

10. X. Hu et al., "Unlearning Implicit Social Biases During Sleep," *Science* 348, no. 6238 (May 29, 2015): 1013–1015, https://doi.org/10.1126/science.aaa3841.

11. Background on NEXTUP from interviews with Robert Stickgold and Antonio Zadra. Also see Antonio Zadra and Robert Stickgold, *When Brains Dream: Understanding the Science and Mystery of our Dreaming Minds* (New York: W.W. Norton & Company, 2021), 108–129.

Chapter Eight: Life Unfiltered

1. Charlotte Beradt, *The Third Reich of Dreams*, trans. Adriane Gottwald (Chicago: Quadrangle Books, 1966), 5.

2. Beradt, *Third Reich of Dreams*, 9.

3. Beradt, *Third Reich of Dreams*, 17.

4. Magdalena J. Fosse et al., "Dreaming and Episodic Memory: A Functional Dissociation?" *Journal of Cognitive Neuroscience* 15, no. 1 (January 1, 2003): 1–9, doi: 10.1162/089892903321107774.

5. For information on Hall/Van de Castle norms, see "Normative Tables for the Hall/Van de Castle Coding System," Dreambank.net, https://dreams.ucsc.edu/Norms/index.html.

6. Calvin S. Hall, "A Cognitive Theory of Dream Symbols," *Journal of General Psychology* 49 (1953): 273–282, https://doi.org/10.1080/00221309.1953.9710091.

7. Calvin S. Hall, "Diagnosing Personality by the Analysis of Dreams," *Journal of Abnormal and Social Psychology* 42, no. 1 (1947): 68–79, https://doi.org/10.1037/h0054344.

8. Hall, "Cognitive Theory of Dream Symbols": 169–186.

9. Beradt, *Third Reich of Dreams*, 8.

10. For background on the continuity hypothesis including the case of Karl, see G. William Domhoff, "Dreams Are Embodied Simulations That Dramatize Conceptions and Concerns: The Continuity Hypothesis in Empirical, Theoretical, and Historical Context," *International Journal of Dream Research* 4, no. 2 (October 2011): 50–62.

11. G.W. Domhoff, *Dreaming as the Embodiment of Thoughts: A Widower's Dreams of His Deceased Wife*, paper presented to the annual meeting of the Association for Psychological Science, Chicago, Illinois (2008).

12. Domhoff, *Dreaming as the Embodiment of Thoughts*.

13. D. Foulkes, *Dreaming: A Cognitive-Psychological Analysis* (Hillsdale, NJ: Lawrence Erlbaum, 1985). For background on the work of David Foulkes, see G. William Domhoff, *The Scientific Study of Dreams: Neural Networks, Cognitive Development, and Content Analysis* (Wash-

ington, DC: APA Press, 2002), https://dreams.ucsc.edu/TSSOD/The_Scientific_Study_of
_Dreams_2003.pdf.

14. Quotations and background on the study, see Richard N. Wolman and Miloslava Kozmová, "Last Night I Had the Strangest Dream: Varieties of Rational Thought Processes in
Dream Reports," *Consciousness and Cognition* 16, no. 4 (2007): 846 and 838–849.

15. T. L. Kahan and S. P. LaBerge, "Dreaming and Waking: Similarities and Differences Revisited," *Consciousness and Cognition* 20, no. 3 (2011): 509 and 494–514.

16. M. Schredl and A. S. Göritz, "The Frequency of Contacting Persons You Dreamed About:
A Social Aspect of Dreaming," *Imagination, Cognition and Personality* 41, no. 4 (2022):
490–501, https://doi.org/10.1177/02762366221077631.

17. William Dement, *Some Must Watch While Some Must Sleep* (San Francisco: W.H. Freeman
and Company, 1972), 53.

18. Walt Whitman, "Song of Myself, 51," *Leaves of Grass* (New York: Penguin Books, 1959), 85.

19. Kelly Bulkeley, *Big Dreams: The Science of Dreaming and the Origins of Religion* (New York:
Oxford University Press, 2016), 108.

20. Frequency of negative dreams varies across studies. For background on negativity in
dreams, see T. A. Nielsen et al., "Emotions in Dream and Waking Event Reports," *Dreaming* 1, no. 4 (1991): 287–300, https://doi.org/10.1037/h0094340.

21. Rosalind Cartwright and Lynne Lamberg, *Crisis Dreaming: Using Your Dreams to Solve
Your Problems* (New York: HarperPerennial, 1992), 6.

22. Alan B. Siegel, *Dream Wisdom: Uncovering Life's Answers in Your Dreams* (Berkley: Celestial Arts, 2002), 62–88.

23. Carolyn Winget and Frederic T. Kapp, "The Relationship of the Manifest Content of
Dreams to Duration of Childbirth in Primiparae," *Psychosomatic Medicine* 34, no. 4
(July-August 1972): 317.

24. For quotation and background on study, see T. Nielsen and T. Paquette, "Dream-Associated
Behaviors Affecting Pregnant and Postpartum Women," *Sleep* 30, no. 9 (September 2007): 1167
and 1162–1169, doi: 10.1093/sleep/30.9.1162, PMID: 17910388, PMCID: PMC1978400.

25. Cartwright and Lamberg, *Crisis Dreaming: Using Your Dreams to Solve Your Problems*, 5.

Chapter Nine: The Power of Big Dreams

1. Excellent background on how the dreaming brain operates in a different mode and the
"real" experiences of dreams from interviews with Michael Schredl and M. Schredl, *Researching Dreams: The Fundamentals* (Switzerland: Palgrave Macmillan, 2018).

2. For background on impactful dreams, see D. Kuiken and S. Sikora, "The Impact of Dreams
on Waking Thoughts and Feelings," in *The Functions of Dreaming*, ed. A. Moffitt, M.
Kramer, and R. Hoffmann (Albany: State University of New York Press, 1993), 419–476;
D. Kuiken et al., "The Influence of Impactful Dreams on Self-Perceptual Depth and Spiritual Transformation," *Dreaming* 16, no. 4 (2006): 258–279, https://doi.org/10.1037/1053
-0797.16.4.258.

3. Harrison S. Chow et al., "Anesthetic-Induced Intraoperative Dream Associated with Remission of a Psychiatric Disorder: A Case Report," *A&A Practice* 16, no. 8 (August 2022), https://doi.org/10.1213/xaa.0000000000001613.

4. W. Alexander et al., "Pharmacotherapy for Post-Traumatic Stress Disorder in Combat Veterans," *Pharmacy and Therapeutics* 37, no. 1 (January 2012): 32–38.

5. U.S. Department of Veteran Affairs, *PTSD: National Centre for PTSD*, February 3, 2023, https://www.ptsd.va.gov/understand/common/common_adults.asp#:~:text=Women percent20arepercent20morepercent20likelypercent20to,sexualpercent20assaultpercent E2percent80percent94comparedpercent20topercent20men.

Chapter Ten: The Power of Little Dreams

1. Excellent background on the process of dreaming, see M. Schredl, *Researching Dreams: The Fundamentals* (Switzerland: Palgrave Macmillan, 2018).

2. For background on Elsewhere AI's Freudian and Jungian interpretation modes, see Kelly Bulkeley's summaries: https://interpret.elsewhere.to/en/styles/freudian/ and https://interpret.elsewhere.to/en/styles/jungian/.

3. Descriptions of both Freudian and Jungian interpretations were generated using Elsewhere AI.

4. Descriptions are from the interpretations generated by Elsewhere AI.

5. For background on dream journaling and its prevalence among groups, see M. Schredl, *Analyzing A Long Dream Series: What Can We Learn About How Dreaming Works?* (New York: Routledge, 2024).

6. For a detailed account of the Barb Sanders case study including dream series, interviews, and analysis, see W. G. Domhoff, "Barb Sanders: Our Best Case Study to Date, and One That Can Be Built Upon," Dreamresearch.net, https://dreams.ucsc.edu/Findings/barb_sanders.html.

7. For quotation and background on Montague Ullman's work and method, see M. Ullman and N. Zimmerman, *Working with Dreams* (New York: Delacorte Press, 1979), 13.

8. Ullman and Zimmerman, *Working with Dreams*. For more information on dream salons, visit dreamsid.com. My dream is displayed on the gallery page along with other dreams painted by Julia Lockheart.

9. M. Schredl, "Sharing Dreams: Sex and Other Sociodemographic Variables," *Perceptual and Motor Skills* 109 (2009): 235–238, https://doi.org/10.2466/pms.109.1.235-238.

10. K. Ijams and L. D. Miller, "Perceptions of Dream-Disclosure: An Exploratory Study," *Communication Studies* 51, no. 2 (2000): 135–148, https://doi.org/10.1080/10510970009388514.

11. M. Schredl and J. A. Schawinski, "Frequency of Dream Sharing: The Effects of Gender and Personality," *American Journal of Psychology* 123, no. 1 (2010): 93–101, https://doi.org/10.5406/amerjpsyc.123.1.0093.

12. M. R. Olsen, M. Schredl, and I. Carlsson, "Sharing Dreams: Frequency, Motivations, and Relationship Intimacy," *Dreaming* 23, no. 4 (2013): 245–255, https://doi.org/10.1037 /a0033392.

13. M. Schredl et al., "Emotional Responses to Dream Sharing: A Field Study," *International Journal of Dream Research* 8, no. 2 (2015): 135–138, https://doi.org/10.11588 /ijodr.2015.2.23052.

14. M. Blagrove. and J. Lockheart, *The Science and Art of Dreaming* (New York: Routledge, 2023), 143.

15. For background on storytelling and artistic virtuosity and sexual selection, see G. Miller, *The Mating Mind: How Sexual Choice Shaped the Evolution of Human Nature* (New York: Doubleday and Co., 2000); D. Smith et al., "Cooperation and the Evolution of Hunter-Gatherer Storytelling," *Nature Communications* 8, no. 1 (2017): 1853, https://doi .org/10.1038/s41467-017-02036-8, PMID: 29208949, PMCID: PMC5717173. For background on the possible evolutionary function of dreams, see M. Blagrove, "Does Dreaming Have a Function?" *Psychologist*, The British Psychological Society, March 15, 2024, https://www.bps.org.uk/psychologist/does-dreaming-have-function.

16. For background on the empathy theory of dreaming, see M. Blagrove et al., "Testing the Empathy Theory of Dreaming: The Relationships Between Dream Sharing and Trait and State Empathy," *Frontiers in Psychology* 10 (2019): 1351, https://doi.org/10.3389 /fpsyg.2019.01351, PMID: 31281278, PMCID: PMC6596280.

17. For background on the relationship between empathy and fiction, see P. M. Bal and M. Veltkamp, "How Does Fiction Reading Influence Empathy? An Experimental Investigation on the Role of Emotional Transportation," *PLOS ONE* 8, no. 1 (2013): e55341, https://doi.org/10.1371/journal.pone.0055341; K. Oatley, "Fiction: Simulation of Social Worlds," *Trends in Cognitive Sciences* 20, no. 8 (2016): 618–628, https://doi.org/10.1016/j .tics.2016.06.002.

Chapter Eleven: Dream Odyssey

1. For excellent resources and background on lucid dreaming, visit Stephen LaBerge's The Lucidity Institute website at lucidity.com.

2. K. R. Konkoly et al., "Real-Time Dialogue Between Experimenters and Dreamers During REM Sleep," *Current Biology* 31, no. 7 (2021): 1418, https://doi.org/10.1016/j .cub.2021.01.026.

3. Konkoly et al., "Real-Time Dialogue," 1419.

4. Descriptions of German, Dutch, French lucid dreaming experiments from Konkoly et al., "Real-Time Dialogue," 1417–1427 and e6.

5. Konkoly et al., "Real-Time Dialogue," e4.

6. Aristotle, *On Dreams*, trans. J. I. Beare (350 BC), https://classics.mit.edu/Aristotle/dreams.html.

7. St. Augustine. (AD 415), *The Letters Of St. Augustine*, Letter 159.

8. Hervey de Saint-Denys, *Les Rêves et les Moyens De Les Diriger: Observations Pratiques* (Dreams and the Ways to Direct Them: Practical Observations), ebook, eds. Carolus den Blanken and Eli Meijer, 2016 (Paris: Amyot, 1867), 7.

9. F. van Eeden, *A Study of Dreams* (1913), https://www.dreamscience.ca/en/documents /Newpercent20content/lucidpercent20dreamingpercent20pdfs/vanEeden_PSPR_26_1 -12_1913.pdf.

10. S. LaBerge, *Lucid Dreaming: The Power of Being Awake & Aware in Your Dreams* (New York: Ballantine Books, 1985), 41.

11. LaBerge, *Lucid Dreaming,* 42

12. K. Hearne, *The Dream Machine: Lucid Dreams and How to Control Them* (Little Falls, NJ: The Aquarian Press, 1990), 11.

13. B. Baird e al., "Episodic Thought Distinguishes Spontaneous Cognition in Waking from REM and NREM Sleep," *Conscious Cognition* 97 (January 2022): 103247, doi: 10.1016 /j.concog.2021.103247.

14. M. Dresler et al., "Neural Correlates of Dream Lucidity Obtained from Contrasting Lucid Versus Non-lucid REM Sleep: A Combined EEG/fMRI Case Study," *SLEEP* 35, no. 7 (2012): 1017–1020.

15. A. Gilboa, "Autobiographical and Episodic Memory—One and the Same? Evidence from Prefrontal Activation in Neuroimaging Studies," *Neuropsychologia* 42, no. 10 (2004): 1336–1349.

16. D. T. Saunders et al., "Lucid Dreaming Incidence: A Quality Effects Meta-analysis of 50 Years of Research," *Consciousness and Cognition* 43 (2016): 197–215, https://doi.org /10.1016/j.concog.2016.06.002.

Chapter Twelve: Dream Engineering: The Next Frontier

1. Kimberley C. Patton, "'A Great and Strange Correction': Intentionality, Locality, and Epiphany in the Category of Dream Incubation," *History of Religions* 43, no. 3 (February 2004): 194–223, https://doi.org/10.1086/423399.

2. K. C. Fox et al., "Dreaming as Mind Wandering: Evidence from Functional Neuroimaging and First-Person Content Reports," *Frontiers in Human Neuroscience* 7 (2013): 412, https://doi.org/10.3389/fnhum.2013.00412; G. W. Domhoff and K. C. Fox, "Dreaming and the Default Network: A Review, Synthesis, and Counterintuitive Research Proposal," *Consciousness and Cognition* 33 (May 2015): 342–353, https://doi.org/10.1016/j.concog.2015.01.019.

3. Thomas Andrillon et al., "Does the Mind Wander When the Brain Takes a Break? Local Sleep in Wakefulness, Attentional Lapses, and Mind-Wandering," *Frontiers in Neuroscience* 13 (September 13, 2019), https://doi.org/10.3389/fnins.2019.00949.

4. Célia Lacaux et al., "Sleep Onset Is a Creative Sweet Spot," *Science Advances* 7, no. 50 (December 10, 2021): eabj5866, https://doi.org/10.1126/sciadv.abj5866.

5. Adam Haar Horowitz et al., "Targeted Dream Incubation at Sleep Onset Increases Post-sleep Creative Performance," *Scientific Reports* 13, no. 1 (May 15, 2023), https://doi.org/10.1038/s41598-023-31361-w.

6. Horowitz et al., "Targeted Dream Incubation at Sleep Onset Increases Post-Sleep Creative Performance."

7. Célia Lacaux et al., "Sleep Onset Is a Creative Sweet Spot," 1.

8. S. Mednick, "The Associative Basis of the Creative Process," *Psychological Review* 69 (1962): 220–232, https://doi.org/10.1037/h0048850.

9. For detailed explanation of the NEXTUP model of why we dream, see Antonio Zadra and Robert Stickgold, *When Brains Dream: Understanding the Science and Mystery of our Dreaming Minds* (New York: W.W. Norton & Company, 2021), 108–129.

10. From conversations with Deirdre Barrett; D. Barrett, "The 'Committee of Sleep': A Study of Dream Incubation for Problem Solving," *Dreaming* 3, no. 2 (1993): 115–122, https://doi.org/10.1037/h0094375.

11. Anat Arzi et al., "Olfactory Aversive Conditioning During Sleep Reduces Cigarette-Smoking Behavior," *Journal of Neuroscience* 34, no. 46 (November 12, 2014): 15382–15393, https://doi.org/10.1523/jneurosci.2291-14.2014.

12. "Spend Saturday Night Dreaming with Zayn Malik: Coors Light and Coors Seltzer Entice Chill and Refreshing Dreams," *Business Wire*, February 4, 2021, https://www.businesswire.com/news/home/20210204005955/en/CORRECTING-and-REPLACING-Spend-Saturday-Night-Dreaming-With-Zayn-Malik.

13. C. Charney and R. Kawles, "Did Covid Kill the Techlash? Future of Marketing Study 2021," https://www.amanewyork.org/wp-content/uploads/2021/10/AMA-NY-Future-of-Marketing-Study-Did-Covid-Kill-the-Techlash.pdf (accessed February 17, 2025).

14. The Pokémon Company, "20 Million Downloads Worldwide!," June 26, 2024, https://www.pokemonsleep.net/en/news/3135303038343737313739343333836393435/#:~:text=2024percent2F6percent2F26-,20percent20Millionpercent20Downloadspercent20Worldwide!,giftspercent20topercent20celebratepercent20thispercent20milestone; Sophie McEvoy, "Pokemon Sleep Surpasses $120M in Revenue," GamesIndustry.biz, September 24, 2024, https://www.gamesindustry.biz/pokemon-sleep-surpasses-120m-in-revenue.

15. NPR, "The Smart Audio Report," 2018, https://www.nationalpublicmedia.com/uploads/2020/04/The-Smart-Audio-Report-Spring-2018.pdf.

16. B. Kinsella, "Yes. The Bedroom Is Now the Most Popular Location for Smart Speakers. Here's Why and What It Means," Voicebot.ai, April 30, 2020, https://voicebot.ai/2020/04/30/yes-the-bedroom-is-now-the-most-popular-location-for-smart-speakers-heres-why-and-what-it-means/.

17. American Academy of Sleep Medicine, "One in Three Americans Have Used Electronic Sleep Trackers, Leading to a Changed Behavior for Many," 2023, https://aasm.org/one-in-three-americans-have-used-electronic-sleep-trackers-leading-to-changed-behavior-for-many/.

18. For background and examples on the dangers of dream advertising, see A. Haar Horowitz, R. Stickgold, and A. Zadra, "Inside Your Dreamscape," *Aeon*, November 19, 2021, https://aeon.co/essays/dreams-are-a-precious-resource-dont-let-advertisers-hack-them.

19. Sizhi Ai et al., "Promoting Subjective Preferences in Simple Economic Choices During Nap," *eLife* 7 (December 6, 2018), https://doi.org/10.7554/elife.40583.

20. Hélène Tanguay et al., "Relationship Between Drug Dreams, Affect, and Craving During Treatment for Substance Dependence," *Journal of Addiction Medicine* 9, no. 2 (March 2015): 123–29, https://doi.org/10.1097/adm.0000000000000105.

21. Federal Communications Commission, March 9, 2001, https://transition.fcc.gov/eb/Orders/2001/da01643.html.

22. 15 U.S.C. § 45 Section 5 of the FTC Act, https://www.federalreserve.gov/boarddocs/supmanual/cch/200806/ftca.pdf.

23. From conversation with Deidre Barrett. For background, also see D. Barrett, "A Reflection on the Letter, 'Advertising in Dreams Is Coming: Now What?,'" *Medium*, February 4, 2021, https://deirdrebarrettdreams.medium.com/dream-incubation-and-adventures-in-ad-land-4f2ca7057ffd.

24. S. Moutinho, "Are Advertisers Coming for Your Dreams? Scientists Warn of Efforts to Insert Commercials into Dreams," *Science*, June 11, 2021, https://www.science.org/content/article/are-advertisers-coming-your-dreams.

25. Elaine Li and Jared Wicker worked on the campaign. For background, see https://www.elaine.li/coors-dream; R. Green, "Q&A with DDB Sydney's Elaine Li and Jared Wicker, Creatives Behind Coors' 'Dream Study' Campaign," *Campaign Brief*, February 8, 2021, https://campaignbrief.com/qa-with-ddb-sydneys-elaine-li-and-jared-wicker-creatives-behind-coors-dream-study-campaign/.

26. D. Marlan, "The Nightmare of Dream Advertising," *William & Mary Law Review* 65, no. 2 (November 2, 2023): 259–326, https://scholarship.law.wm.edu/cgi/viewcontent.cgi?article=4005&context=wmlr.

27. R. Stickgold, A. Zadra, and A. Haar, "Advertising in Dreams is Coming: Now What?," *Dream Engineering*, 2021, https://dxe.pubpub.org/pub/dreamadvertising.

28. Wunderman Thompson, "Trend #39 Dreamvertising," *Wunderman Thompson's Future 100*, 2022, https://www.vml.com/de/campaign/trend-39-from-100-wunderman-thompsons-future-100-trends-2022.

Chapter Thirteen: Conclusion: The Interoception of Dreams

1. For background on interoception, see Carrie DeJong, "Interoception: Our Real-Life Superpower," TEDx Chilliwack, May 5, 2022, video, 14:00, https://www.youtube.com/watch?v=JGnt7L8KVXY. Also see C. M. Schmitt, S. Schoen, "Interoception: A Multi-Sensory Foundation of Participation in Daily Life," *Front Neurosci.* 16:875200 (June 9, 2022).

A Dreamer's Toolkit

1. Célia Lacaux et al., "Sleep Onset Is a Creative Sweet Spot," *Science Advances* 7, no. 50 (December 10, 2021): eabj5866, https://doi.org/10.1126/sciadv.abj5866. For background on Adam Haar and colleagues' sleep onset study, see A. H. Horowitz et al., "Targeted Dream Incubation at Sleep Onset Increases Post-Sleep Creative Performance," *Scientific Reports* 13, no. 1 (May 15, 2023): 7319, https://doi.org/10.1038/s41598-023-31361-w. For background on Salvador Dalí's slumber with a key method, see Salvador Dalí, *50 Secrets of Magic Craftsmanship* (1948).

2. Stephen LaBerge, Keith LaMarca, and Benjamin Baird, "Pre-Sleep Treatment with Galantamine Stimulates Lucid Dreaming: A Double-Blind, Placebo-Controlled, Crossover Study," *PLOS ONE* 13, no. 8 (2018): e0201246, https://doi.org/10.1371/journal.pone.0201246. For background on MILD and lucid dreaming, see Stephen LaBerge, *Lucid Dreaming: A Concise Guide to Awakening in Your Dreams and in Your Life* (Sounds True, 2009); Stephen LaBerge, *Lucid Dreaming: An Exploratory Study of Consciousness During Sleep* (PhD diss., Stanford University, 1980); Daniel Love, "Mnemonic Induction of Lucid Dreaming (MILD)," accessed November 26, 2024, https://www.thelucidguide.com/techniques/mnemonic-induction-of-lucid-dreaming-(mild).

3. Robert Naiman, "Dreamless: The Silent Epidemic of REM Sleep Loss," *Annals of the New York Academy of Sciences* 1406, no. 1 (October 2017): 77–85, https://doi.org/10.1111/nyas.13447.

4. C. V. O. Witvliet, "Forgiveness, Embodiment, and Relational Accountability: Victim and Transgressor Psychophysiology Research," in *Handbook of Forgiveness*, 2nd ed., eds. E. L. Worthington and N. Wade (New York, NY: Brunner-Routledge, 2020), 167–177; also see C. V. O. Witvliet, S. L. Blank, and A. J. Gall, "Compassionate Reappraisal and Rumination Impact Forgiveness, Emotion, Sleep, and Prosocial Accountability," *Frontiers in Psychology* 13 (November 17, 2022): 992768, https://doi.org/10.3389/fpsyg.2022.992768.